£53

Medical and Surgical Diseases of the Pancreas

Medical and Surgical Diseases of the Pancreas

Edited by

Jorge E. Valenzuela, M.D., F.A.C.P., F.A.C.G.
Professor of Medicine
GI/Liver Division
Department of Medicine
University of Southern California School of Medicine
Los Angeles, California

Howard A. Reber, M.D.
Professor and Vice Chairman
Department of Surgery
UCLA School of Medicine
Los Angeles, California
and
Chief, Surgical Service
Sepulveda, VA Medical Center
Sepulveda, California

André Ribet
Professeur Emérite
d'Hépato-gastro-entérologie
Université Paul Sabatier
et
INSERM U151
C.H.U. de Ranqueil
Toulouse, France

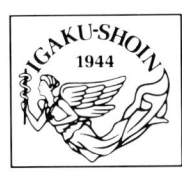

IGAKU-SHOIN New York • Tokyo

Published and distributed by

IGAKU-SHOIN Medical Publishers, Inc.
One Madison Ave., New York, N.Y. 10010

IGAKU-SHOIN Ltd.,
5-24-3 Hongo, Bunkyo-ku, Tokyo

Copyright © 1991 by IGAKU-SHOIN Medical Publishers, Inc.
All rights reserved. No part of this book may be translated or reproduced in any form by print, photo-print, microfilm or any other means without written permission from the publisher.

Library of Congress Cataloging-in-Publication Data

Medical and surgical diseases of the pancreas / edited by Jorge E. Valenzuela, Howard A. Reber, and André Ribet.
p. cm.
Includes bibliographical references and index.
1. Pancreatitis. 2. Pancreas—Surgery. I. Valenzuela, Jorge E.
[DNLM: 1. Pancreatitis—physiopathology. 2. Pancreatitis—surgery. WI 805 M489]
RC858.P35M43 1991
616.4'6—dc20
DNLM/DLC
for Library of Congress 91-4656
CIP

ISBN: 0-89640-180-4 (New York)
ISBN: 4-260-14180-5 (Tokyo)

Printed and bound in the U.S.A.

10 9 8 7 6 5 4 3 2 1

Preface

In the last decade, there have been considerable advances in our knowledge of the cell biology and physiology of the pancreas. Our understanding of the possible pathogenetic mechanisms of pancreatitis also has improved markedly. Concurrently new diagnostic and therapeutic procedures have modified and improved the medical and surgical management of patients with pancreatic diseases.

This book was written as a practical review of the basic mechanisms of diseases, with emphasis in problem solving examples, and practical use of the physiological basis of diseases. Also included are areas that cover GI hormones, endocrine and exocrine pancreas, diagnostic tests—including ERCP, ultrasound, CT, and MRI, acute and chronic pancreatitis, complications, and cancer.

We hope to provide the practicing physician, as well as medical students, residents, and practicing gastroenterologists, with a simplified update of new developments in the daily management of patients with pancreatic problems.

To my wife, Elena Valenzuela.
To my parents, Louis and Rose Reber.

Contributors

Joel W. Adelson, M.D., Ph.D.
Director, Division of Pediatric
 Gastroenterology and Nutrition
Rhode Island Hospital
and
Professor of Pediatrics and Physiology
Brown University
Providence, Rhode Island

Hartley Cohen, M.D., F.A.C.G.
Associate Professor of Clinical
 Medicine
Chief of LAC—USC Medical Center
 Endoscopy Unit
GI/Liver Diseases Division
Department of Medicine
University of Southern California
 School of Medicine
Los Angeles, California

H. Gill Cryer, M.D., Ph.D.
Assistant Professor of Surgery
Director, Trauma Emergency Surgery
 Service
UCLA Medical Center
Los Angeles, California

David A. Goldstein, M.D.
Associate Professor and Chief
Division of General Internal Medicine
Co-Director, Pacific Center for Health
 Policy and Ethics
University of Southern California
 School of Medicine
Los Angeles, California

James H. Grendell, M.D.
Associate Professor of Medicine and
 Physiology
University of California, San Francisco
Chief, Gastroenterology Section
San Francisco V.A. Medical Center
San Francisco, California

Nariman D. Karanjia, FRCS
Registrar in Surgery
London, England
and
Research Fellow
Department of Surgery
UCLA School of Medicine
Los Angeles, California

Laurence Leichman, M.D.
Associate Professor of Medicine
Division of Oncology
Los Angeles County—University of
 Southern California Medical Center
Los Angeles, California

Jacques Moreau, M.D.
Practicien Hospitalier
 au C.H.R. de Toulouse
Service de Gastro-entérologie
 et Nutrition
C.H.U. de Ranqueil
Toulouse, France

Philip W. Ralls, M.D.
Associate Professor, Radiology
Chief, Section of Body Imaging and
  Interventional Radiology
Los Angeles County—University of
  Southern California Medical Center
Los Angeles, California

Howard A. Reber, M.D.
Professor and Vice Chairman
Department of Surgery
UCLA School of Medicine
Los Angeles, California
and
Chief, Surgical Service
Sepulveda, VA Medical Center
Sepulveda, California

André Ribet
Professeur Emérite
d'Hépato-gastro-entérologie
Université Paul Sabatier
et
INSERM U151
C.H.U. de Ranqueil
Toulouse, France

Jorge E. Valenzuela, M.D., F.A.C.P., F.A.C.G.
Professor of Medicine
GI/Liver Division
Department of Medicine
University of Southern California
  School of Medicine
Los Angeles, California

Nancy E. Warner, M.D.
Hastings Professor
Department of Pathology
University of Southern California
  School of Medicine
Los Angeles, California

Russell Yang, M.D., Ph.D.
Assistant Professor of Medicine
Associate Director, Clinical GI Training
GI/Liver Diseases Division
Department of Medicine
University of Southern California
  School of Medicine
Los Angeles, California

Contents

1. Pancreatic Physiology   1
   Jorge E. Valenzuela

2. Classification and Pathology of Acute Pancreatitis   23
   Nancy E. Warner
   Howard A. Reber

3. Pathogenic Mechanisms of Pancreatitis   29
   Jorge E. Valenzuela
   André Ribet

4. Clinical Presentation of Acute Pancreatitis   47
   Howard A. Reber
   Jorge E. Valenzuela
   Hartley Cohen

5. Imaging Studies in Acute Pancreatitis   61
   Philip W. Ralls

6. Management of Acute Pancreatitis   67
   Jorge E. Valenzuela

7. Local Complications of Pancreatitis Including Pseudocyst and Ascites   73
   Howard A. Reber
   H. Gill Cryer

8. Systemic Complications of Acute Pancreatitis   87
   James H. Grendell
   David A. Goldstein

9. Chronic Pancreatitis   99
   André Ribet
   Jacques Moreau
   Jorge E. Valenzuela

10. Diagnosis of Chronic Pancreatitis   113
    André Ribet
    Jacques Moreau
    Jorge E. Valenzuela

11. Radiology in Chronic Pancreatitis   125
    Philip W. Ralls
    Hartley Cohen

12. Treatment of Chronic Pancreatitis   131
    André Ribet
    Jacques Moreau
    Jorge E. Valenzuela
    Howard A. Reber
    Nariman D. Karanjia

13. Pancreatic Disease in Infants and Children   143
    Joel W. Adelson

14. Carcinoma of the Exocrine Pancreas   155
    Russell Yang
    Laurence Leichman
    Philip W. Ralls
    Hartley Cohen
    Nariman D. Karanjia
    Howard A. Reber

Index   179

Medical and Surgical Diseases of the Pancreas

Chapter 1
Pancreatic Physiology

JORGE E. VALENZUELA

The exocrine pancreas secretes between 6 and 20 g of proteins per day and is the main source of hydrolytic enzymes, which play a major role in the digestion of nutrients in the intestine. The amount of enzymes secreted greatly exceeds the hydrolytic capacity necessary for an ordinary meal.

The aim of this chapter is to review current concepts of the function of the exocrine pancreas. The characteristics of pancreatic juice, the physiology of the secretory cells, and the mechanisms that regulate pancreatic secretion are analyzed. Whenever possible the information provided will be related to human physiology. When this is impossible, concepts will refer to animal models.

PANCREATIC JUICE

The pancreas secretes an alkaline isotonic solution rich in electrolytes and enzymes. The anions are mainly bicarbonate and chloride. The sum of these anions is relatively constant at about 150 mmol/L. The concentration of bicarbonate varies directly with the flow rate. At maximal rate of secretion, bicarbonate concentration may be close to 140 mmol/L. The high bicarbonate content of pancreatic juice regulates intraintestinal pH by buffering the acidic content of gastric juice that is delivered into the duodenum.

Pancreatic juice contains more than 20 different proteins, most of which have actual or potential enzyme activity. Proenzymes and enzymes include three forms of trypsinogen; two forms each of procarboxypeptidase A and B; two proelastases and chymotrypsinogens (only one in human juice); and one form each of procolipase, amylase, lipase, and carboxyl-ester hydrolase, and prophospholipase A_2.[1]

Proteolytic Enzymes

Pancreatic proteases, with gastric proteases, degrade dietary proteins into amino acids and oligopeptides necessary for absorption. In addition, trypsin activates other pancreatic enzymes by hydrolysis of proenzymes.

Depending on the site of activity, the proteolytic enzymes can be divided into endopeptidases (ie, trypsinogens, chymotrypsinogens, and elastases) with specificity for peptides at the interior of the protein chain, and exopeptidases (ie, carboxypeptidases) that preferentially split C-terminal bonds of the peptides, thus complementing the action of endopeptidases.

Trypsinogens

Three forms of the proenzyme trypsinogen have been identified in human pancreatic juice: a cationic trypsinogen, an anionic form, and an intermediate form. Their molecular weights (MW) range between 26,000 and 28,000 and their catalytic activities are similar. There is twice as much cationic trypsinogen as anionic trypsinogen, and very small quantities of the intermediate or mesotrypsinogen. Overall trypsinogens represent more than 20% of the total proteins of human pancreatic juice.

Under normal conditions, including the presence of calcium, trypsinogens are readily activated by an enteropeptidase (enterokinase), present in the brush border of the duodenal mucosa. This enteropeptidase ruptures the lysine–isoleucine bond of trypsinogen and releases active trypsins. After this initial activation, trypsins undergo an autoactivation process. The total amount of active trypsin in the lumen of the intestine is limited by autolysis, which takes place at pH 8. This autolysis is limited by the presence of Ca^{2+}, which in concentrations greater than 1 mM stabilizes the zymogens.

Soybean trypsin inhibitor has different effects on the different trypsinogens. Whereas anionic trypsin is completely inhibited, cationic trypsin is only partially inhibited by equimolar quantities of the inhibitor. The intermediate form or mesotrypsin shows no inhibition.[2]

Chymotrypsinogen

Two molecular forms of chymotrypsinogen (MW 24,000 to 27,000 d) have been identified in human pancreatic juice and constitute approximately 13% of the total proteins of pancreatic juice. This endopeptidase is activated by trypsin and has limited specificity for aromatic bonds like those next to phenylalanine, tyrosine, and tryptophan.

Carboxypeptidases

Two procarboxypeptidases, A and B, have been identified in human pancreatic juice. They have similar molecular weights of approximately 47,000, and activation of the proenzymes seems to occur after a large peptide is freed, resulting in an active enzyme with a MW of approximately 34,000.

Carboxypeptidases A are exopeptidases that contain one Zn^{2+} per molecule and hydrolyze bonds next to an α-carboxyl C-terminal. This enzyme has preferential activity for aromatic structures but is also active on neutral or acid structures.

Two carboxypeptidases B with similar MW but with the B2 form carrying more negative charges have been isolated from human pancreatic juice. These exopeptidases are active on basic C-terminal aminoacids and complement the digestive actions of trypsin and carboxypeptidases A. Carboxypeptidase B has been identified in the islets of Langerhans, which suggest this enzyme may play a role in the metabolism of insulin.

Two proelastases found in human pancreatic juice represent about 5% of the protein. These enzymes are unique because they degrade elastin, a component of blood vessels and lung, and have been implicated in the pathogenesis of both emphysema and the vascular damage observed in some cases of pancreatitis. Human proelastase 1 is anionic and has a MW of approximately 29,000, whereas proelastase 2 is cationic and has a lower MW of 25,000. Both proenzymes are activated by trypsin, and when active they are completely inhibited by the serum protease inhibitors α1-antitrypsin and α2-macroglobulin.

Small quantities of pancreatic ribonucleases, deoxyribonucleases, and kallikreinogen can be identified in human pancreatic fluid. Their physiologic significance remains unknown.

The trypsin inhibitor (Kazal inhibitor) has been isolated from pure pancreatic juice. It is a basic polypeptide with a molecular weight of 6242 d that represents about 1% of the total protein of the human pancreatic juice. It is secreted in the free form; effectively inhibits human cationic trypsin by forming an inactive, relatively stable complex; and its concentration in pancreatic juice is sufficient to inhibit up to 20% of the potentially active trypsin. This trypsin inhibitor is one of the most important factors in preventing trypsinogen activation and autodigestion of the pancreas. In chronic alcoholics the ratio of trypsin to trypsin inhibitor is increased, perhaps accounting for the increased incidence of pancreatitis in this population.[3]

Elevated levels of circulating pancreatic secretory trypsin inhibitor have been observed in some cases of acute pancreatitis. This elevation may persist for several days. Measuring this inhibitor in the blood may have diagnostic value.

Lipolytic Enzymes

Human pancreatic juice contains one lipase that exists as two isoenzymes. It has a MW of about 48,000 and isoelectric points of 6.5. This makes pancreatic lipase distinct from salivary and gastric lipase, which are stable at acid pH and have an optimal pH between 2.5 and 6.5. In fact, when an excess of acid enters the duodenum, as occurs in gastrinoma, pancreatic lipase is inhibited and denatured, resulting in impaired lipid hydrolysis and steatorrhea. The main substrate for pancreatic lipase are triglycerides present at the hydrophobic–hydrophilic phases. The enzyme is specific for primary ester bonds in the 1 and 3 positions of triglycerides. The hydrolysis leads to sequential production of diglycerides, monoglycerides, and fatty acids. Bile salts present in the intestine cause a physical separation of lipase from its substrate by increasing surface pressure. This effect is reversed by colipase.

Colipase, secreted as a proenzyme and activated by tryptic digestion, enhances lipase activity in the presence of bile salts. Colipase has a low MW of about 10,000, has a high affinity for phospholipid-covered surfaces, and seems to form a complex with lipase that binds to the substrate, even at high surface pressure.

The human pancreas also secretes carboxyl ester lipase, also called cholesterol lipase. This is a glycoprotein with a MW of about 100,000, an optimal pH of 8.0, and a broad substrate specificity. This enzyme, in the presence of trihydroxy bile salts, hydrolyzes cholesterol in the intestine.

Prophospholipase A2 activity is found in human pancreatic juice. This zymogen must be activated by trypsin, yielding an N-terminal heptapeptide. The active enzyme has a MW of approximately 14,000 and an optimal pH of 8.5. In the presence of bile and calcium it splits fatty acid ester bonds at the 2 position. Phospholipase A_2 generally can attack membrane phospholipids with hydrolysis of some of their components (such as lecithin), generating lysolecithin, which is cytotoxic. Increased phospholipase A_2 and lysolecithin levels have been found in necrotic tissue and exudate of patients with pancreatitis, fostering speculation that this enzyme could play a role in the pathogenesis of pancreatitis.[4]

Amylolytic Enzymes

Although some digestion of carbohydrates begins in the mouth, pancreatic amylase plays a major role in the digestion of starch. The pancreas secretes large quantities of an alpha amylase which specifically hydrolases the 1–4 links of amylase and amylopectin, producing oligosaccharides and dextrins. The oligosaccharides undergo further hydrolysis by specific oligosaccharidases at the intestinal membrane surface. The amount of amylase secreted by the pancreas exceeds that needed to accomplish carbohydrate digestion after a standard meal. Malabsorption of carbohydrates is rarely a clinical problem, even when exocrine function is markedly impaired, because of the presence of salivary amylase, the stability of this enzyme, and the presence of brush-border hydrolases. There is evidence that wheat flour contains a protein that inhibits more selectively salivary amylase. It is probable that this protein is normally destroyed by gastric juice.

Lysosomal Enzymes

Human pancreatic juice also contains small amounts of some acidic lysosomal hydrolases. Lysosomal enzymes are mainly large glycoproteins that can be bound to the inner aspect of the lysosomal membrane. Their main role is to degrade extracellular material like secretagogues after internalization, and endogenous cellular constituents. In the latter case, the process is referred to as "autophagy." Lysosomes can also degrade excess secretory material, a function known as "crinophagy." Lysosomes can secrete digested or undigested materials, and also lysosomal enzymes by exocytosis to the lumen of the duct. The secretion in the human pancreatic juice of some of these enzymes, for example, N-acetyl-β-D-glucosaminidase, arylsulfatase, N-acetyl-β-D-galactosaminidase, α-L-fucosidase, and α-D-mannosidase, increases after administration of cholecystokinin (CCK), in a way similar to the digestive enzymes. In contrast, another group of lysosomal enzymes, including β-D-glucoronidase, leucine naphthylamidase, and α-D-glucosidase, do not increase consistently after CCK administration.[5] Lysosomal enzymes, because of their low concentration, low optimal pH, and instability in the intestinal lumen, probably do not play an important role in the digestion of nutrients. They appear to have a role in the degradation of ligands after internalization and the disposal of degraded cellular constituents, however.

Other proteins, for example, small amounts of gamma glutamyl transferase, alanine transaminase, and alkaline phosphatase, have been identified in pancreatic juice. The determination of these enzymes in pancreatic juice has been attempted for diagnostic purposes. Results have been disappointing, however. Lactoferrin is an iron-binding protein present in acinar cells that is secreted in small amounts into the pancreatic juice of healthy subjects. Lactoferrin concentration increases significantly in the juice of patients with chronic calcifying pancreatitis.

Low levels of carcinoembryogenic antigen (CEA), CA 19–9, and α-fetoprotein activities have been detected in pure pancreatic juice from healthy subjects. The concentration of these proteins may increase in patients with chronic pancreatitis, and an additional increase may occur in patients with pancreatic cancer. Measurement of these peptides in pure pancreatic juice as a diagnostic test for pancreatic cancer has not become widely used, however, due to its low sensitivity and specificity.

Acid extracts of pancreas and human pancreatic juice have yielded a protein with a MW of approximately 14,000 that prevents formation of insoluble calcium salts. It has been named pancreatic stone protein (PSP). PSP is decreased in the pancreatic juice of patients with chronic alcoholic pancreatitis and appears to play a pathogenic role in the formation of pancreatic calculi.[6]

Less than 2% of the proteins of human pure pancreatic juice are serum proteins. These proteins probably reach the pancreatic ducts through the intercellular spaces, but the relatively high concentration of immunoglobulin A (IgA) suggests that the pancreas synthesizes the secretory component of the dimeric IgA. The concentration of these enzymes is not altered by CCK or cholinergic stimulation. Serum protein concentration in the juice of patients with calcifying pancreatitis is increased, probably due to altered permeability. Some peptides, for example, somatostatin, insulin, glucagon, and CCK, can be found in pancreatic juice. The relatively high concentration of these peptides in the juice suggests a nonplasmatic origin, but their regulation and role in pancreatic secretion remain unknown.

PHYSIOLOGY OF PANCREATIC SECRETORY CELLS

The acinus is the basic unit of the exocrine pancreas. Acini are grouped in secretory lobules of about 5 mm in diameter that are separated by connective tissue septa. The acinar cells have a characteristic morphology, with a truncated, pyramidlike shape surrounding the lumen of the acinus, which is lined by the centroacinar cells (Fig. 1.1). The juice secreted by the acini flows into intralobular ducts, which empty into interlobular ducts, which drain into the pancreatic duct.

Pancreatic secretion originates from two cells of the exocrine pancreas, the acinar cell and the centroacinar cell. The acinar cell synthesizes and releases secretory en-

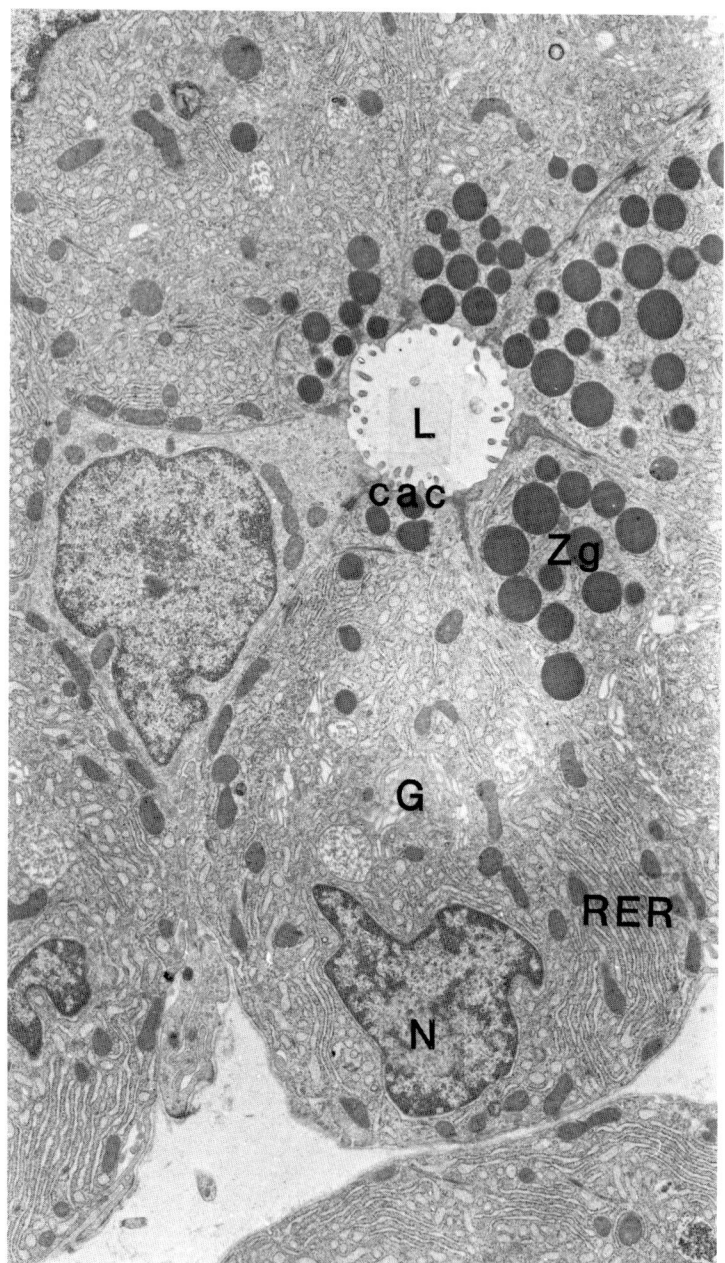

FIGURE 1.1. Micrograph of a monkey acinus depicting the acinar lumen (L), one centroacinar cell (cac), acinar cell nucleus (N), rough endoplasmic reticulum (RER), zymogen granules (Zg) and the Golgi complex (G) ($\times$ 4850) (Courtesy of Dr. Richard Wood).

zymes and fluid with a composition similar to that of the plasma, whereas the centroacinar cell secretes water and electrolytes.

Acinar Cells

Polarity is an important characteristic of acinar cells. Hormones (ligands) bind with receptors at the basolateral membrane, whereas protein secretion normally takes place at the luminal membrane. The basolateral membrane also contains guanosine triphosphate (G) proteins and *effectors*, which translate the stimulus to intracellular messengers that ultimately activate the secretory process. Several *receptors* have been identified at the basolateral membrane, where they interact with specific regulators such as CCK, bombesin, vasoactive intestinal peptide (VIP), secretin, acetylcholine, and somatostatin in a process called stimulus–secretion coupling. Coupling leads to interaction with the G proteins of the membrane, which in turn activate effector enzymes or open ion channels in the cell (Fig. 1.2). Effectors are compounds such as 1,2,diacylglyceride (DAG) or enzymes such as phospholipase C (PLC), phosphatidylinositol phosphodiesterase (PI-Pase), or adenylcyclase (AC), which serve as vectors to transmit information across the cell membrane to the cytoplasm. These processes not only regulate the secretory process but also affect cell metabolism, growth, and gene expression.

Studies on the molecular mechanisms of secretagogues have centered on two distinct pathways, the calcium pathway and the cyclic adenosine monophosphate (cAMP) pathway.[7]

The Calcium Pathway

The calcium pathway process is activated by binding of muscarinic agents, cholecystokinin, gastrin, bombesin, litorin, physalaemin, substance P, and eledoisin to specific receptors. This binding mobilizes cellular calcium and after a series of steps stimulates enzyme secretion. The process is probably initiated by activation of phospholipase C, which is associated with the cytoplasmic phase of the plasma membrane and reacts with phosphorylated derivatives of phosphatidylinositol (PI). Hydrolysis of PI bisphosphate (PIP 2) results in the formation of two compounds that function as intracellular messengers. One compound is Inositol 1,4,5-triphosphate (Ins-1,4,5-P3), which mobilizes calcium from stores inside the cell by opening Ca^{2+} channels, possibly in the endoplasmic reticulum (ER). The pool of free calcium in the cytosol increases with activation of calcium–calmodulin-dependent protein kinases that are ultimately responsible for exocytosis. The increased level of Ca^{2+} in the cytoplasm is transient as Ca^{2+} channels open with Ca^{2+} efflux from the cell. Sustained secretion is dependent on extracellular Ca^{2+}, with probable direct activation of protein kinase C and possible generation of arachidonic acid. During this process of activation, there also is increase in the intracellular levels of cyclic guanosine monophosphate (cGMP), the function of which is unknown. The second compound generated by phospholipase C is diacylglycerol (DAG), a poorly soluble compound that activates protein kinase C (see Fig. 1.2).

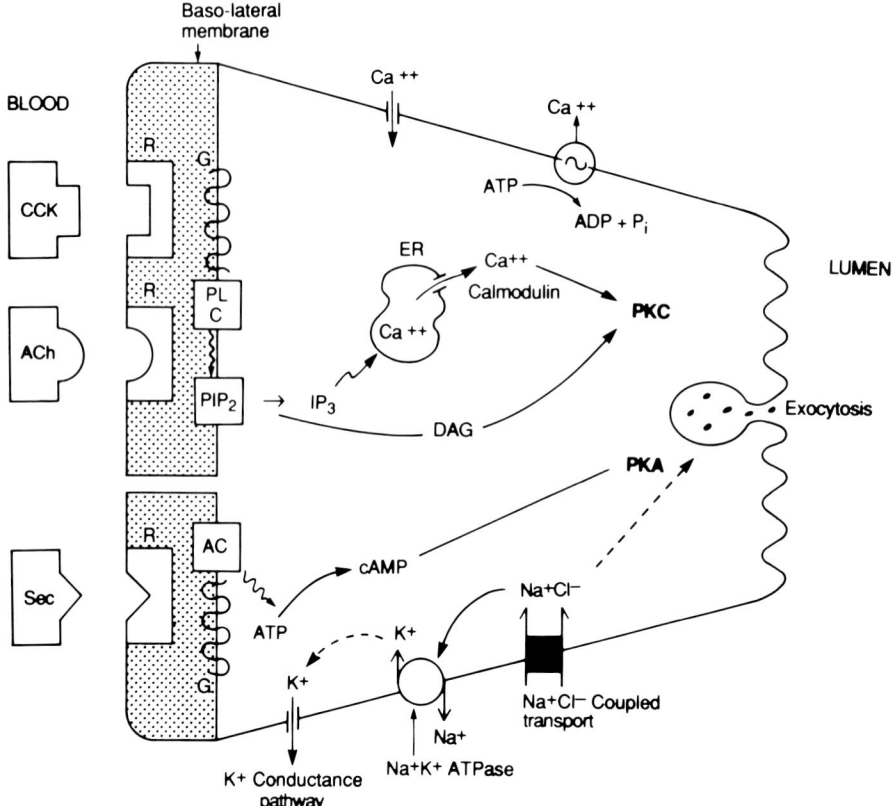

FIGURE 1.2. Illustration of stimulus–secretion coupling at the acinar cell. (CCK, cholecystokinin; Ach, acetylcholine; Sec, secretin; R, receptors for agonists, G, regulatory proteins; PLC, phospholipase C; Ac, adenyl cyclase; cAMP, cyclic adenosine monophosphate; PIP2, phosphatidyl-inositol disphosphate; IP3, inositol triphosphate; ER, endoplasmic reticulum; DAG, diacylglycerol; PKC, protein kinase C; PKA, protein kinase A.)

In addition, the binding of secretagogues, similar to the binding of CCK or acetylcholine to the acinar cell, depolarizes the basolateral membrane by an extracellular Ca^{2+}-dependent mechanism, which results in opening of channels selective for anions and cations. Activation of Na^+K^+ ATPase pumps in the basolateral membrane facilitates K^+ passage in and Na^+ out of the acinar cell. An Na^+Cl^- coupled transport mechanism mediates transport of Na^+ and Cl^- to the cytoplasm, favoring Cl^- secretion at the luminal pole of the cell. Flux of Cl^- at the apical membrane drives net transport of water, which facilitates solubilization and secretion of enzymes (see Fig. 1.2).

The cAMP Pathway

The cAMP pathway system involves binding of secretagogues such as secretin, VIP, and cholera toxin to specific receptors in the acinar cell membrane. This initiates a cascade of events leading to activation of adenyl cyclase and increased formation of intracytosolic cAMP. It is possible that signal transduction in this system involves sequential interaction of the agonists with guanidine nucleotide-binding proteins (Gs), and the adenylate cyclase catalyst (AC).[8] Secretagogues that generate cAMP also stimulate exchange of Na^+ and K^+ by a mechanism that is independent of Ca^{2+} (see Fig. 1.2).

Digestive enzyme secretion ultimately takes place when the intracellular messengers Ca^{2+}, DAG, or cAMP alter the phosphorylation of protein kinases (PK).

Stimulation of both systems results in potentiation, which means the total secretory response is higher than the sum of either individual system alone. The mechanism of this potentiation is unknown.

In addition to enzyme secretion per se, activation of either pathway is accompanied by other cellular processes affecting the secretory enzymes, the first of which is biosynthesis.

Biosynthesis of Secretory Proteins

In general, expression of pancreatic genes occurs through specific proteins that direct the uptake and transport of different peptides toward intracellular compartments, where they will perform specific functions. The expression of the pancreatic genes can be regulated at the transcriptional and translational level either by changes in the concentration of hormones and neurotransmitters, or by alterations in the composition of the diet. For instance, prolonged infusion of a CCK analogue to the rat can induce preferential synthesis of anionic trypsinogen and chymotrypsinogen with a decrease in amylase synthesis. In contrast, infusion of secretin stimulates synthesis of lipase and infusion of insulin stimulates synthesis of amylase.

Secretory digestive enzymes and lysosomal enzymes are synthesized on ribosomes as large polypeptides containing short-lived terminal signal peptides recognizable by receptors in the rough ER (RER) membrane. Recognition facilitates translocation of the polypeptide chain across the RER membrane to the intracisternal space. During this process the signal peptide is cleaved, leaving the protein bound to the internal aspect of the RER. From this compartment the proteins are transferred sequentially to the *cis*-face of the Golgi complex and to the condensing vacuoles (immature granules). From there the secretory proteins are sorted by specific protein carriers to the zymogen granules and the lysosomal enzymes are transported to lysosomes. During stimulation by secretagogues, the content of the zymogen granules is discharged by exocytosis, which involves fusion of the zymogen granule membrane with the luminal membrane of the apical portion of the acinar cell, and release of the enzymes to the central acinar lumen.

Initial studies revealed that the different proteins maintain a relatively fixed proportion in fasting conditions and after stimulation. This led to the concept that the secretory proteins are secreted in parallel or fixed ratios. More recent observations, however, have noted that the proportion of the secretory proteins may vary. This finding has been interpreted in two ways.

According to Scheele, changes in secretory proteins can occur in a coordinate manner, with similar latency and kinetics.[9] This is known as the exocytosis–vectorial transport hypothesis. In other instances, such as those occurring during the transition between fasting and meal-stimulated secretion, the changes are dissimilar and even occur in opposite directions, resulting in anticoordinate responses. During the period of transition, the pancreas can accumulate zymogen granules with different compositions. The pool of proteins could vary if the pancreas is stimulated again, and in this instance the proportion of enzymes could vary as well. In any case, according to this hypothesis, the secretory proteins would not leave at any stage of the secretory process the membrane-bound compartments to which they are attached.[10]

Another interpretation is that there may be at least two secretory pathways in the acinar cell. For instance, it has been noted that basal secretion contains preferentially newly synthesized enzymes. It also has been observed that CCK and its analogues increase secretion of older stored enzymes with relative inhibition of newly synthesized proteins, but ultimately both types of enzymes are secreted. In addition, there is evidence that cholinergic stimulation increases release of old enzymes while it inhibits release of newly synthesized proteins. These different responses have been interpreted as evidence for alternative sources of enzymes within the cell, including an extragranular source.[11] An additional alternative interpretation is that there are different populations of granules, which differ in their enzyme composition.

Various pathways can respond differently to differing secretagogues. A cytoplasmatic extragranular route has been observed in other cells, with enzymes either transported freely through the cytoplasm or in microvesicles. If this last phenomenon occurs in the acinar cell, it is possible that the cytoplasmic pool of enzymes is in equilibrium with the enzymes of the zymogen granules, and eventually also in equilibrium with the extracellular space. This hypothesis challenges the concept that the membrane of the zymogen granule is impermeable to its contained secretory proteins, and implies that there is exchange of enzymes between the granule and the cytoplasm. Secretion of enzymes would result from direct transport of individual proteins across the membranes by diffusionlike processes.[12]

Small quantities of pancreatic enzymes also can be detected in the peripheral blood, and there is evidence that blood levels of certain proteases such as cationic trypsinogen increase after a meal. These enzymes may leak back from the pancreatic ducts, although it has been proposed that they represent a form of endocrine secretion of enzymes through the basolateral membrane of the acinar cells.[13]

In conclusion, it is evident that, in the acinar cell, all aspects of biosynthesis, storage, transport, and secretion of enzymes have not been fully resolved. It is possible that clarification of these intracellular events may help to elucidate the mechanism of premature enzyme activation, which is believed to be crucial in the pathogenic mechanisms of pancreatitis.

Centroacinar and Duct Cells

Centroacinar cells are situated between acinar cells and occupy the center of the acinus (see Fig. 1.1). The same type of cells line the intralobular ducts and the smaller interlobular ducts. Ductal cells are the source of pancreatic bicarbonate, and participate in the exchange of chloride. At the acinus the secretion from the acinar cells is rich in Cl^-, and secretions from the centroacinar cells are rich in HCO_3^-. The final concentration of these electrolytes in the juice delivered to the duodenum is determined by passive exchange of HCO_3^- for Cl^- in the ductal system as the juice courses to the intestine.

There is a variety of mechanisms that stimulate electrolyte and water secretion, and there are remarkable differences between different species regarding the volume and composition of basal cells and the rate of postpranidial secretion.

The cellular events that take place in the centroacinar and ductal cell during stimulation are similar to those that occur in the acinar cell. Secretagogues, including peptides, catecholamines, and acetylcholine, bind to specific receptors in the cell membrane with either release of bound guanosine diphosphate (GDP) from inactive G protein, with subsequent activation of adenylate cyclase, or increase in intracellular concentration of Ca^{2+}. Secretin, VIP, and related peptides stimulate secretion by increased concentration of cAMP. Secretin is about 10 times more potent than VIP. The available information suggests that Ca^{2+} plays no role in the action of secretin. The intracellular steps after increased cytosolic cAMP generation in the centroacinar cell are unknown.

High bicarbonate content in pancreatic juice is achieved by nonionic diffusion at the small duct and centroacinar cells. Inside these cells bicarbonate is in equilibrium with carbonic acid, which is in equilibrium with protons and CO_2. Protons are translocated through the basolateral membrane to the interstitial fluid by a Na^+H^+ exchanger, whereas carbonic acid and CO_2 diffuse through the cell basolateral membrane. Bicarbonate becomes trapped and a conducting channel in the apical membrane drives bicarbonate into the lumen. Na^+ is believed to diffuse passively through the paracellular route, whereas water is driven by osmotic pressure.

Chloride concentration is inversely related to the rate of pancreatic flow and is determined by exchange with bicarbonate through the excretory ducts. Sodium concentration in pancreatic juice is about 160 mmol, which is higher than in plasma, whereas concentration of potassium is similar to that of plasma. Although it has been proposed that both ions enter the juice passively through the paracellular route, replacement of either ion on the serosal side decreases the rate of fluid secretion, suggesting that both cations participate by an indirect mechanism in the control of the secretory process.

Pancreatic juice also contains small quantities of calcium that appear to originate from acinar cells. Calcium is secreted with enzymes and by passive diffusion across the epithelium. An alkaline secretion rich in electrolytes reaches the duodenum and serves to buffer the gastric acidic content delivered to the duodenum. There is no evidence that pancreatic bicarbonate secretion is decreased in patients with duodenal ulcer, although it has been observed that smoking, an aggravating factor in ulcers, decreases bicarbonate secretion and lowers intraduodenal pH.

CONTROL OF PANCREATIC SECRETION

Food ingestion is the most important stimulant for pancreatic secretion. In humans as well as in other species, however, there is a small but discernible amount of pancreatic juice secreted between meals, known as interdigestive or basal secretion.

Interdigestive Pancreatic Secretion

A small volume of pancreatic secretion with low HCO_3^- content and about one tenth the enzyme output observed after a meal can be measured in humans during the interdigestive pattern. This secretion shows cyclic variations that are related to phases of the migrating motility complex (MMC), however.

These variations of interdigestive pancreatic secretion were originally described in the dog by Boldyreff in 1911, and have been better defined in the last decade by simultaneous motility recordings and secretory measurement in humans.[14] Three phases can be identified: The first phase of the cycle is characterized by motor quiescence, and low volume of gastric acid and pancreatic secretions. During phase II there is increasing and irregular motor activity in the stomach and intestine, whereas pancreatic secretion increases in volume and enzyme content. Concomitantly, secretion of bile into the duodenum also increases, possibly due to cyclic contraction of the gallbladder. During phase III there is a burst of peristaltic activity that affects the stomach, duodenum, jejunum, and ileum sequentially while gastric acid secretion peaks, pancreatic enzyme secretion is maintained at the level of phase II, and bicarbonate secretion reaches the highest interdigestive level. After phase III motility and secretions return to the low levels of phase I. The overall duration of the cycle is approximately 90 minutes in humans, with considerable variations between individuals and during the day and night. Phase I lasts 10 to 20 minutes, phase III 5 to 8 minutes, and the rest of the cycle corresponds to phase II (Fig. 1.3).

The mechanism responsible for the control of interdigestive pancreatic secretion remains unknown. Based on animal studies, however, there is evidence that vagotomy and superior mesenteric ganglionectomy suppress the cyclic changes of basal pancreatic secretion. Plasma levels of two peptides, motilin and pancreatic polypeptide (PP), also show cyclic variations that suggest some participation in this mechanism. For instance, motilin blood levels peak during phases II and III, and exogenous administration of this peptide initiates motor activity in the gastroduodenal segment with a pattern similar to phase III. Administration of exogenous motilin to produce blood levels similar to those occurring during phase III does not affect pancreatic secretion in humans, however. In addition, the initiating of phase III beyond the gastric level is not related to changes in blood levels of motilin. Plasma levels of PP also peak during phase III, but this peptide is an inhibitor of pancreatic secretion. In conclusion, a hormonal role for the interdigestive cyclic secretory pattern remains undetermined.

Pancreatic Secretory Response to a Meal

Anticipation, tasting, and swallowing of food elicits a potent pancreatic secretory response that usually exceeds the needs for normal digestion of the nutrients in an average meal. The magnitude of the enzyme secretion has been determined in humans and varies with the volume, consistency, and composition of the meal. Studies from the Mayo Clinic comparing a homogenized meal with a solid–liquid meal found that basal enzyme secretion increased about 5-fold with both meals, although the

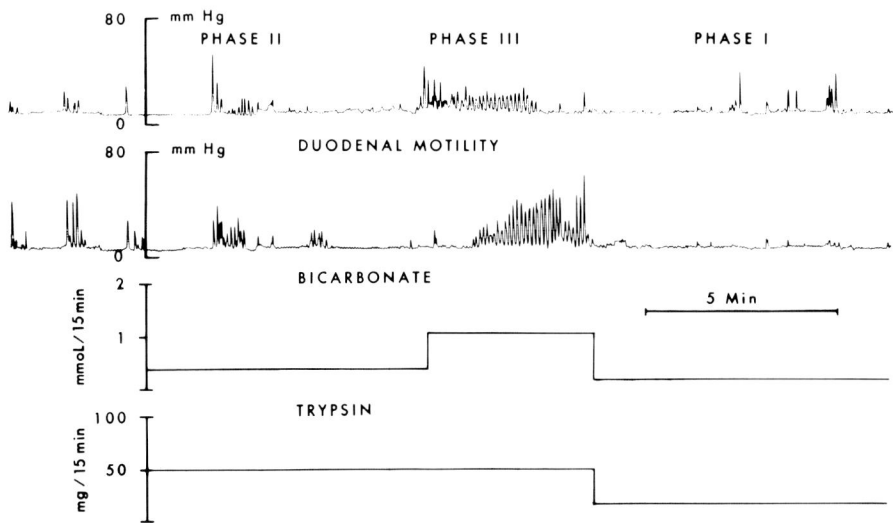

FIGURE 1.3. Representative tracing of the interdigestive duodenal motility, bicarbonate, and trypsin output in duodenal aspirate of a healthy human subject.

duration of the secretory response was longer after the solid meal.[15] Overall the increased enzyme secretion lasts for about 5 hours. All chemical constituents of food are able to stimulate the pancreas, although fat and proteins are the most potent. The mechanisms that participate in the control of the pancreatic response to a meal are mediated by neural and hormonal pathways, with both stimulatory and inhibitory impulses. These impulses initiate, maintain, and suppress pancreatic secretion as long as food particles are present in the intestine.

Although the secretory response to food ingestion represents a coordinated interaction at different levels, these mechanisms are divided according to the level of origin as the cephalic, gastric, and intestinal phases. The different phases frequently overlap, share pathways, and eventually can replace each other, as occurs after total gastrectomy or truncal vagotomy.

Cephalic Phase of Pancreatic Secretion

Anticipation, smell, sight, mastication, and probably contact of the food with the pharynx and esophagus stimulate the cephalic phase of pancreatic secretion in humans. If acid is prevented from entering the duodenum, there is minimal bicarbonate secretion and the overall enzyme response amounts to about 50% of the response to a meal. Without gastric aspiration, which allows gastric secretion to trigger intestinal mechanisms, secretion of bicarbonate rises and the enzyme response reaches near maximal levels. This response is abolished by vagotomy, whereas atropine markedly suppresses the secretion of enzymes but does not alter bicarbonate secretion.[16] From this it may be concluded that vagal cholinergic pathways mediate the cephalic phase of enzyme secretion, whereas noncholinergic, possibly peptidergic pathways, participate in the bicarbonate response. The putative transmitter for this last effect has not been fully identified, but VIP is the most likely candidate. This peptide, contained in nerves that are close to the pancreatic ducts, is released after electric vagal stimulation, and in experimental animals antiserum against VIP suppresses the secretory reponse to vagal stimulation.[17] There is no evidence that the cephalic phase alters the plasma levels of peptides such as gastrin, secretin, or CCK.

There is little information regarding the neuromodulation of pancreatic secretion at the central nervous system (CNS) level. Several peptides may be involved, as in gastric secretion and gastrointestinal motility. A study shows that intracerebroventricular injection of thyrotropin-releasing hormone (TRH) stimulates pancreatic enzyme secretion. This effect is blocked by vagotomy, whereas TRH shows no effect when injected intravenously.[18]

There is no evidence of an inhibitory component in the cephalic phase of pancreatic secretion in humans, although sham-feeding (a common method to study cephalic stimulation) releases PP, a peptide that inhibits pancreatic enzyme secretion.

Gastric Phase of Pancreatic Secretion

The presence of food in the stomach affects pancreatic secretion by direct pathways, and indirectly stimulates acid secretion that in turn elicits duodenal stimulatory impulses. Both mechanisms can be activated by gastric distention and chemically-mediated release of peptides. Distention of a balloon in the stomach of humans increases flow and pancreatic enzyme secretion. This response is suppressed by atropine, and after vagotomy there is a prolonged period of inhibition. This can be taken as evidence that the pancreatic secretory response is mediated by a cholinergic gastropancreatic vagovagal reflex, although there is weak evidence that some release of gastrin could take place. Gastrin is released when products of protein digestion reach the antral mucosa, and some stimulatory effect of relatively high doses of gastrin on human pancreatic enzyme secretion has been described. A physiologic role for gastrin on human pancreatic secretion is not firmly established. However, gastrin alone probably has a weak stimulatory effect on pancreatic enzyme secretion in humans. It is possible that, acting in concert with neural reflexes and other peptides released by the intestine, gastrin may contribute to the overall pancreatic response to a meal.

Studies in healthy subjects show that when a balanced meal is placed in the stomach, there is a strong pancreatic enzyme response with about a 5-fold increase in enzyme secretion. This response lasts for about 5 hours (Fig. 1.4). The relative contribution of the gastric phase to the overall postprandial pancreatic secretory response has not been quantitated, but it seems to be moderate. Some estimate of this can be made by examining the abnormalities in pancreatic secretion occurring in patients after antrectomy or gastrectomy. It is difficult to separate the direct effect of gastric resections from the effects on other functions of the stomach affected by surgery, however, including inhibition of acid secretion, abnormal trituration of solid meals, and partial digestion of proteins and fats by the stomach. The latter effects may interfere indirectly by affecting intestinal stimulatory mechanisms of pancreatic secretion.

There is no clear evidence of an inhibitory component in the gastric phase of pancreatic secretion in humans, although food in the stomach also releases PP, which is a known inhibitor of pancreatic secretion.

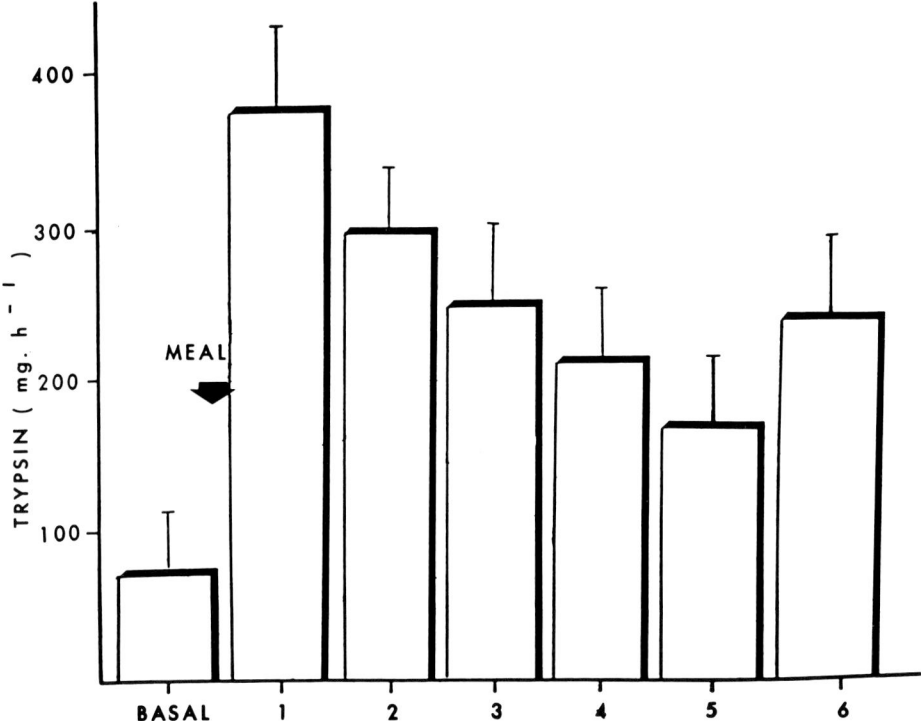

FIGURE 1.4. Mean (± SEM) trypsin output in six volunteers during basal and after intragastric administration of a liquid meal.

Intestinal Phase of Pancreatic Secretion

When it reaches the intestine, chyme triggers the most important mechanisms that affect pancreatic secretion. These mechanisms are neural and hormonal, and have stimulatory and inhibitory effects on the pancreas. The interaction between these excitatory and inhibitory impulses explains why the pancreatic secretory response after administration of exogenous hormones is greater than that elicited by a meal.

STIMULATORY NEURAL MECHANISMS IN THE INTESTINE

Increasing the volume or osmolality of duodenal content causes a modest increase in pancreatic flow and enzyme secretion without detectable changes in the plasma levels of secretin or CCK. Atropine prevents this response, so it is assumed that this effect is mediated by cholinergic duodenopancreatic reflexes.[19] Experiments with transplanted pancreas confirm that the presence of aminoacids in the intestine stimulates pancreatic secretion through a double pathway, one mediated by nerves and another mediated by the release of hormones.[20]

Muscarinic receptors have been identified in the acinar cells. Furthermore, there is evidence that cholinergic agents increase levels of cytosolic Ca^{2+} in the acinar cell with activation of kinases involved in the exocytosis. There is evidence that adrenergic nerves can stimulate amylase secretion directly, independent from blood flow changes. There is also evidence that this effect is mediated by an adrenergic receptor and uses cAMP as intracellular messenger. The presence of other peptides in the pancreatic nerve terminals has been documented, and they may play a role in the mechanisms that control pancreatic secretion. In addition to VIP, immunoreactivity to PHI, a 27-amino acid peptide related to VIP; CCK; gastrin-releasing peptide (GRP); bombesin; enkephalins; neuropeptide Y (NPY); and somatostatin have been detected in pancreatic nerves. Some of these peptides, for example, somatostatin, may also have a paracrine effect (action by release to the neighborhood of the target cell) on the exocrine pancreas. It is not known how these peptides participate in the enteropancreatic reflexes. There is no clear evidence for an inhibitory neural mechanism at the intestinal level for pancreatic enzyme secretion.

Stimulatory Intestinal Hormonal Mechanisms

The hormones secretin and CCK play a key role in the control of the intestinal phase of pancreatic secretion. Secretin is released primarily in the proximal small intestine by hydrogen ions with a pH threshold of 4.0 to 4.5. Fatty acids and bile salts also release secretin from the intestinal mucosa independently from low duodenal pH. Secretin is a potent stimulant of bicarbonate and enzyme secretion. Basal plasma secretin levels of 2 to 4 pg/mL as measured by specific radioimmunoassay rise to 8 pg/mL after a meal (Fig. 1.5), and there is significant correlation between this plasma secretin increment and pancreatic bicarbonate secretion.[21] In addition, secretin stimulates enzyme secretion.

Secretin release is not affected by vagotomy or atropine, but the pancreatic bicarbonate response is decreased by both. Conversely, there is experimental evidence that vagal stimulation in certain species stimulates bicarbonate secretion. This effect is only partially suppressed by atropine or adrenergic blockers, suggesting that other neurotransmitters may be involved in this response. The relatively small increment in plasma secretin, and the considerable amount of bicarbonate that is secreted postprandially, suggest that interaction with other hormones like CCK, VIP, and neurotensin, or neural pathways potentiate the stimulatory effect of secretin on ductular cells.

CCK, a potent stimulant of pancreatic enzyme secretion, also is released primarily in the proximal small intestine by fatty acids, oligopeptides, certain l-isomers of amino acids (phenylalanine and tryptophan), glucose, and nonalcoholic components of beer. Preventing contact of pancreatic proteolytic enzymes with duodenal mucosa increases plasma CCK levels further, suggesting that pancreatic proteases play a negative regulatory mechanism on CCK release.

Several molecular forms of CCK with similar molar potencies have been identified in plasma (CCK-8, CCK-33, CCK-39, CCK-58. It is possible that CCK is released

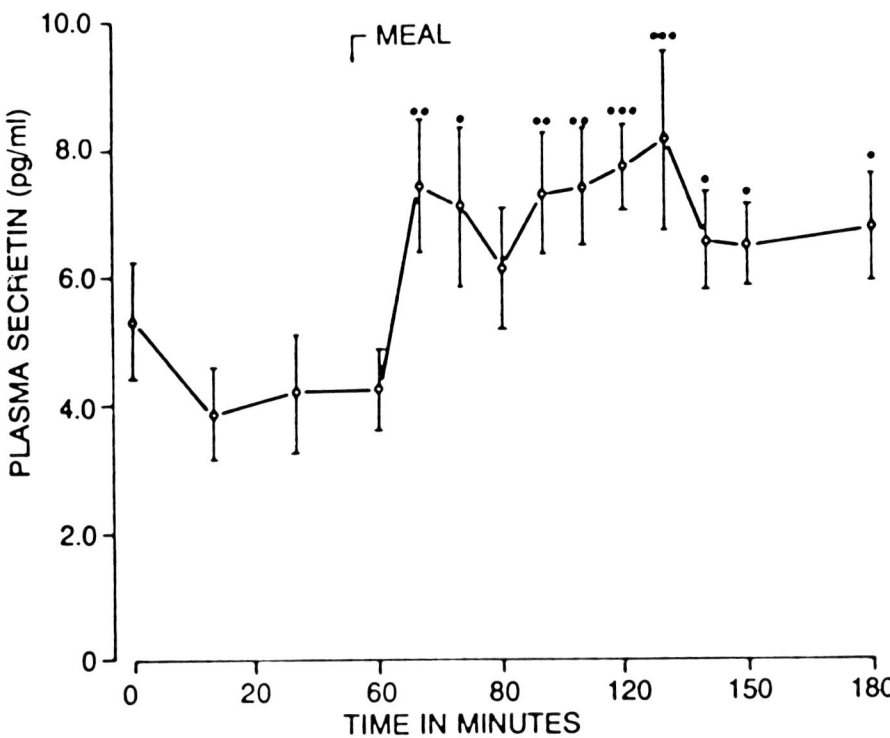

FIGURE 1.5. Mean (± SEM) plasma secretin concentrations after fasting and a standard meal in healthy subjects. Values after the meal (asterisks) were significantly different from basal values. (From Chey WY, et al. Plasma secretin and pancreatic secretion in response to liver extract meal with varied pH and exogenous secretin in the dog. *Am J Physiol* 1982; 324:263–272.

as a large precursor molecule that undergoes some degradation in the circulation. Using specific radioimmunoassays and one bioassay, low plasma CCK levels have been measured at 1 to 2 pM during fasting. After a meal, plasma CCK levels increase to 120 to 160 pg/mL measured by radioimmunoassay and 10 to 12 pM measured by bioassay. At these plasma levels, CCK appears to have a potent stimulatory effect on acinar cells. After administration of L364,718, a potent and specific CCK antagonist, a decrease by about 60% of the pancreatic enzyme response to a meal has been observed in experimental animals.[22] From these studies we may conclude that CCK alone is responsible for more than half the postprandial enzyme secretory response. The present evidence shows that neither CCK release nor enzyme secretion in response to exogenous CCK are affected by atropine or vagotomy.

Bombesin, a tetradecapeptide isolated from amphibian skin, and gastrin releasing peptide (GRP) also play a role in the control of human pancreatic secretion. Bombesinlike immunoreactivity is present in the pancreas. Moreover, exogenous administration of bombesin stimulates release of gastrin (bombesin has structural similarities with GRP) and CCK. Additionally, GRP and bombesin directly stimulate amylase secretion from dispersed pancreatic acinar cells from human pancreas.[23]

Other peptides such as VIP and neurotensin also stimulate pancreatic secretion of bicarbonate and enzymes. VIP seems to be a weak stimulant, however, and it is unlikely to play a significant role in the secretory response to food in humans. Neurotensin plasma levels increase in humans after a fatty meal, and supraphysiologic doses of neurotensin stimulate secretion of bicarbonate and enzymes. A firm role for this peptide in the overall postprandial pancreatic response in humans has not been established, however. In general, interpretation of results after exogenous administration of peptides such as VIP, neurotensin, and others (peptide YY, neuropeptide Y) is compounded by their effects on pancreatic blood supply and their ability to interact with CCK receptors on vagal nerve fibers. A complex interaction of these peptides on blood flow and parasympathetic activity is becoming evident.

Insulin seems to have important metabolic and secretory effects on acinar cells. For instance, insulin potentiates the effect of CCK or cholinomimetics on enzyme secretion. Protein synthesis seems to be insulin dependent. The role of insulin on acinar function may explain the decreased secretory capacity of the pancreas in diabetics.

Intestinal Hormonal Inhibitory Mechanisms

Pancreatic polypeptide (PP) is a polypeptide consisting of 36 amino acids (MW 4200), and is released by endocrine cells of the pancreas in response to vagal cholinergic pathways initiated by stimulation at the cephalic level (sham feeding in humans), the gastric level (gastric instillation of a nutrient), and in the small intestine. CCK plays the most important role in the release of PP since high levels of PP are observed after administration of exogenous CCK, whereas postprandial PP release is inhibited by CCK antagonists. Plasma PP levels show a biphasic increase after a meal, and a role for this peptide in the modulation of pancreatic secretion is suggested by the observation that exogenous administration of PP to mimic postprandial PP plasma levels inhibits pancreatic secretion. Because there are no receptors for PP in the acinar cell, and PP affects neither the secretion of the isolated perfused pancreas nor dispersed rat acinar cells, it is assumed that PP effects are mediated by intermediate neural pathways.

Somatostatin

This peptide is present in the D cells of islets in the pancreas and may reach the exocrine pancreas through the insuloacinar portal circulation or through systemic blood. Plasma levels of somatostatin increase after a meal. Two molecular forms with 14 and 28 amino acids have been identified. Somatostatin is a potent inhibitor of pancreatic bicarbonate and enzyme secretion in humans. In addition, somatostatin inhibits the release of secretin, PP, insulin, and glucagon. Vagal electric stimulation decreases somatostatin secretion. From this it may be surmised that somatostatin plays an important modulating role in pancreatic secretion, either directly at the acinar cell or indirectly through nerves or islet cell hormones. The importance of the paracrine role is not clear.[24]

Several other peptides inhibit pancreatic secretion. For instance, exogenous glucagon inhibits pancreatic secretion of bicarbonate and enzymes in humans. Because there is a several-fold increase in glucagonlike immunoreactivity after a meal, it is conceivable that this peptide participates in the modulation of the pancreatic secretory response to meal. It is not known whether this effect is determined by pancreatic glucagon or by related peptides like enteroglucagon or glicentin. Significant quantities of opioid peptides are found in the human pancreas. This may be important because it is known that morphine stimulates water and bicarbonate but inhibits enzyme secretion. An inhibitory effect for endogenous opiates is suggested by the observation that naloxone increases pancreatic secretion in humans.[25] This effect can be mediated by modulating acetylcholine release from nerve terminals, and by direct interaction with CCK, as occurs in other systems.

Calcitonin gene-related peptide (CGRP), a 37 amino acid peptide predicted by analysis of the calcitonin gene-coding sequence, has been localized in endocrinelike or paracrinelike cells and nerve fibers of the pancreas. CGRP inhibits the release of insulin and somatostatin and inhibits pancreatic secretion, suggesting that it plays an endocrine–paracrine role in the modulation of pancreatic function.

A colonic phase of pancreatic secretion has been proposed for many years. Perfusion of oleic acid into the cecum inhibits pancreatic secretion. There seems to be a humoral mediator of this effect. The colon contains an abundance of endocrine cells and there is some evidence that peptide YY (PYY) could be the pancreatone proposed earlier. PYY is structurally related to PP and to a newly isolated neurotransmitter, neuropeptide Y (NPY). PYY is found in high concentrations in the mucosal epithelium of the ileum and colon and is released after perfusion of fat into the distal intestine. Studies in dogs have shown that exogenous PYY inhibits meal-stimulated pancreatic secretion, and that it can also inhibit secretin and CCK-stimulated pancreatic secretion. It was postulated that PYY could be one of the peptides with pancreotone properties. More recent studies show that although exogenous PYY, when achieving plasma levels similar to those observed postprandially, inhibits acid and pepsin secretion of healthy volunteers, it did not inhibit human pancreatic secretion.[26] In summary, although there is conclusive evidence for an inhibitory humoral mechanism on pancreatic secretion when fats are perfused in the ileocolonic mucosa, one yet unidentified peptide could be the real pancreotone. An alternative possibility is that several peptides could play the pancreotone or anti-CCK role. PYY alone does not seem to be responsible for this effect.

Catecholamines influence pancreatic secretion by a dual mechanism. They cause vasoconstriction and they have direct effect on the secretory cells. A similar role seems to be played by NPY, which is found to coexist with norepinephrine in vascular sympathetic nerve endings and in nerve fibers of the parasympathetic division of the autonomic nervous system. A dual role is also postulated for VIP, because VIP fibers can also be demonstrated in blood vessels of the pancreas, and possibly part of the stimulatory effect of VIP on pancreatic secretion could be mediated by vasodilation.

Feedback Regulation of Pancreatic Secretion

In addition to the neural and humoral inhibitory mechanisms of pancreatic secretion, there is evidence that the presence of pancreatic proteases and bile in the

TABLE 1.1. **Summary of Mechanisms of Pancreatic Secretion Response to a Meal**

Stimuli	Level	Pathway	Effect
Anticipation sight, tasting, smelling, swallowing	Cephalic	Vagus (Ach, VIP?)	↑ Enzymes ↑ HCO_3^-
Food in the stomach Distention H^+ sec.	Gastric	Reflexes(Ach, VIP?) Gastrin Secretin PP ?	↑ Enzymes ↑ Enzymes ↑ HCO_3^- ↑ Enzymes and HCO_3^-
Chyme in the intestine	Intestinal		
Stimulatory Distention Acid Proteins Fats	(duodenum and jejunum)	Reflexes(Ach,VIP?) Secretin, VIP CCK S + CCK Bombesin?	↑ Enzymes ↑ HCO_3^- ↑ Enzymes ↑ HCO_3^- and enzymes ↑ Enzymes
Inhibitory Trypsin Chyme Chyme	(duodenum and jejunum) (ileocolonic)	↓ CCK release PP Somatostatin PYY?	↓ Enzymes ↓ Enzymes and HCO_3^- ↓ Enzymes and HCO_3^- ↓ Enzymes

duodenum plays an important role in the regulation of pancratic enzyme secretion. For instance, diversion of pancreatic juice from the intestine is associated with a marked increase in secretion of enzymes and with high plasma levels of CCK. Trypsin inhibitors are strong CCK secretagogues. Conversely, administration of trypsin or other proteases suppresses CCK release and inhibits pancreatic enzyme secretion. These effects appear to be mediated by a CCK-releasing factor that is inactivated by proteases. After a meal, proteins compete for trypsin activity and the CCK-releasing factor becomes free and stimulates release of CCK. The existence of this mechanism has been documented in the rat and there is inconclusive evidence that is present in humans. It has been observed that administration of large amounts of exogenous proteases to some patients with chronic pancreatitis and moderate pancreatic exocrine insufficiency suppresses pancreatic secretion and CCK release and reduces abdominal pain.[27] These data also raise the possibility that patients with chronic pancreatitis may have increased postprandial plasma levels of CCK that would cause excessive secretory stimulation and perhaps increased pancreatic ductal pressure. This hypothesis has not been confirmed, however. In addition, a small peptide called "monitor peptide" (MW 1000 to 5000) has been purified from rat pancreatic juice. It has some structural homology with trypsin inhibitors and causes an increase in CCK concentrations in the portal blood. It is not known whether a similar peptide is present in human pancreatic juice. Bile diversion and administration of cholestyramine also increase significantly the release of CCK and pancreatic enzyme secretion. This suggests that bile salts also play a role in the negative feedback regulation of pancreatic secretion.[28]

In summary (Table 1.1), pancreatic secretory response to a meal is complex, and modulated by stimulatory and inhibitory impulses that originate at cephalic, gastric, and intestinal levels. These impulses can be mediated by hormones or neural pathways, although considerable new information is being gathered that outlines a complex and well-balanced network of pathways. The pancreatic secretory response is the net result of the interaction of these impulses.

References

1. Scheele G, Bartelt D, Bieger W. Characterization of human exocrine pancreatic proteins by two-dimensional isoelectric focusing/sodium dodecyl sulfate gel electrophoresis. *Gastroenterology* 1981;80:461–473.
2. Rinderknecht H, Renner IG, Abramson SB, et al. Mesotrypsin: a new inhibitor-resistant protease in human pancreatic tissue and fluid. *Gastroenterology* 1984;86:681–692.
3. Renner IG, Rinderknecht J, Valenzuela E. Studies of pure pancreatic secretion in chronic alcoholic subjects without pancreatic secretion in chronic alcoholic subjects without pancreatic insufficiency. *Scand J Gastroenterol* 1980;15:241–244.
4. Nevalainen Timo J. The role of phospholipase A in acute pancreatitis. *Scand J Gastroenterol* 1980;15:641–650.
5. Rinderknecht H, Renner IG, Koyama HH. Lysosomal enzymes in pure pancreatic juice from normal healthy volunteers and chronic alcoholics. *Dig Dis Sci* 1979;24:180–186.
6. Guy O, Robles-Diaz G, Adrich Z. Protein content of precipitates present in pancreatic juice of alcoholic subjects and patients with chronic calcifying pancreatitis. *Gastroenterology* 1983;84:102–107.
7. Bruzzone R. The molecular basis of enzyme secretion. *Gastroenterology* 1990;99:1157–1176.
8. Gilman AG. G-proteins: transducers of receptor-generated signals. *Ann Rev Biochem* 1987;56:615–649.
9. Scheele GA. Biosynthesis, segregation, and secretion of exportable proteins by the exocrine pancreas. *Am J Physiol* (Gastrointest. Liver Physiol. 1) 1980;238:G467–G477.
10. Schick, Jurgen, Verspohl R. Two distinct adaptive responses in the synthesis of exocrine pancreatic enzymes to inverse changes in protein and carbohydrate in the diet. *Am J Physiol* (Gastrointest. Liver Physiol. 10) 1984;247:G611–G616.
11. Liebow C. Nonparallel pancreatic secretion: its meaning and implications. *Pancreas* 1988;3:343–351.
12. Rothman SS, Liebow C. Permeability of zymogen granule membrane to protein. *Am J Physiol* 1985;248:G385–G392.
13. Niederau C, Grendell JH. Effects of proglumide on ductal and basolateral secretion of pancreatic digestive enzymes. *Am J Physiol* (Gastrointest. Liver Physiol. 12) 1985;249:G100–G107.
14. Vantrappen GR, Peeters TL, Janssens J. The secretory component of the interdigestive migrating motor complex in man. *Scand J Gastroenterol* 1979;14:663–667.
15. Malagelada Juan-R, Go Vay LW, Summerskill WHJ. Different gastric, pancreatic, and biliary responses to solid-liquid or homogenized meals. *Dig Dis Sci* 1979;24:101–110.

16. Defillipi C, Solomon TE, Valenzuela JE. Pancreatic secretory response to sham feeding in humans. *Digestion* 1982;23:217–223.
17. Holst JJ, Schaffalitzky de Muckadell OB, Fahrenkrug J. Nervous control of pancreatic exocrine secretion in pigs. *Acta Physiol Scand* 1979;105:33–51.
18. Kato Y, Kanno T. Thyrotropin-releasing hormone injected intracerebroventricularly in the rat stimulates exocrine pancreatic secretion via the vagus nerve. *Regul Pep* 1983; 7:347–356.
19. Dooley CP, Valenzuela JE. Duodenal volume and osmoreceptors in the stimulation of human pancreatic secretion. *Gastroenterology* 1984;86:23–27.
20. Singer MV, Solomon TE, Grossman MI. Effect of atropine on secretion from intact and transplanted pancreas in dog. *Am J Physiol* 1980;238:G18–G22.
21. Chey WY, Yang HC, Hendricks JG, et al. Plasma secretin and pancreatic secretion in response to liver extract meal with varied pH and exogenous secretin in the dog. *Am J Physiol* 1982;324:263–272.
22. Konturek SJ, Tasler J, Konturek JW. Effects of non-peptidal CCK receptor antagonist (L-364,718) on pancreatic responses to cholecystokinin, gastrin, bombesin, and meat feeding in dogs. *Gut* 1989;30:110–117.
23. Susini C, Estival A, Scemama JL. Studies on human pancreatic acini: action of secretagogues on amylase release and cellular cyclic AMP accumulation. *Pancreas* 1986; 1:124–129.
24. Debas HT. Somatostatin: physiologic and clinical potential. View Points on Digestive Diseases 1988;20:13–16.
25. Dooley CP, Saad C, Valenzuela JE. Studies of the role of opioids in control of human pancreatic secretion. *Dig Dis Sci* 1988;33:598–604.
26. Adrian TE, Savage AP, Sagor GR. Effect of peptide YY on gastric, pancreatic, and biliary function in humans. *Gastroenterology* 1985;89:494–499.
27. Slaff J, Jacobson D, Tillman CR, et al. Protease-specific suppression of pancreatic exocrine secretion. *Gastroenterology* 1984;87:44—52.
28. Gomez G, Upp JR, Lluis F, et al. Regulation of the release of cholecystokinin by bile salts in dogs and humans. *Gastroenterology* 1988;94:1036–1046.

Chapter 2

Classification and Pathology of Acute Pancreatitis

NANCY E. WARNER
HOWARD A. REBER

Classification of Pancreatitis

Pancreatitis is a nonbacterial inflammation of the pancreas caused by the activation, interstitial liberation, and digestion of the gland by its own enzymes. The clinical severity of an individual episode of pancreatitis varies. There may be only mild abdominal pain for a day or so, and the process can resolve without the need for medical intervention. At the other extreme, an attack may be characterized by severe abdominal and back pain, persistent vomiting, circulatory collapse, and profound disturbances in renal and respiratory function. This can result in death within a few days. Fortunately most episodes are not so severe. Although hospitalization is required, symptoms usually abate within 3 or 4 days, and the overall mortality rate is about 10%. Pancreatitis has been classified into acute and chronic varieties, a distinction that is useful clinically as well as pathogenetically. The original classification[1] has been refined and simplified by several groups of international experts.[2,3]

Acute Pancreatitis

Acute pancreatitis is characterized clinically by acute abdominal pain, elevated concentrations of pancreatic enzymes in blood, and an increase in the quantity of pancreatic enzymes excreted in urine. There may be just a single episode of pancreatitis, or it may recur. In the United States, the most common cause of acute pancreatitis is cholelithiasis.

During a mild attack, the morphologic changes are characterized by pancreatic and peripancreatic edema and fat necrosis, but pancreatic necrosis is absent. This is often referred to as edematous pancreatitis. The mild form may develop into the severe form, or the episode may be severe from the beginning. In severe pancreatitis there is extensive pancreatic and peripancreatic fat necrosis, parenchymal necrosis, and hemorrhage into and around the pancreas. This form of the disease is often referred to as hemorrhagic or necrotizing pancreatitis.

During an episode of acute inflammation, the exocrine and endocrine functions of the gland are impaired for weeks or months. If the cause (eg, cholelithiasis) and any complications (eg, a pseudocyst) of the pancreatitis are eliminated, however, the pancreas is believed to return to normal. Some scarring may persist after a severe attack, but exocrine and endocrine function are normal, and there is little histologic abnormality. Only rarely does acute pancreatitis lead to chronic pancreatitis, even after multiple attacks.

Chronic Pancreatitis

Chronic pancreatitis is characterized clinically by recurrent episodes of abdominal pain indistinguishable from those of acute pancreatitis. Patients may be asymptomatic between episodes, which typically occur 2 or 3 times a year. In most cases, however, the pain-free intervals shorten, and pain may eventually become constant. As the disease progresses pancreatic function becomes impaired. Exocrine insufficiency is manifested by steatorrhea and malabsorption. Endocrine insufficiency causes diabetes, often requiring insulin management. An unusual form of chronic pancreatitis that occurs in about 5% of cases is not associated with pain. In this case pancreatic functional insufficiency is the principle clinical manifestation of the disease. In the United States, the most common cause of chronic pancreatitis is alcoholism.

Chronic pancreatitis is characterized morphologically by a permanent and usually progressive destruction of pancreatic parenchyma. The acinar cells are destroyed first. They are replaced by dense, fibrous scar tissue. Eventually the islet cells are also damaged by this sclerotic process. Often the main pancreatic duct is dilated, sometimes with focal areas of narrowing along its length. Intraductal protein plugs or calculi are common. Both acute and chronic inflammatory cells are present, as well as edema and focal necrosis. Cysts and pseudocysts occur as well.

A distinct morphologic form of chronic pancreatitis is obstructive chronic pancreatitis. Here the ductal system is moderately dilated proximal to the obstruction, most often caused by a tumor or scar from a previous injury. In the obstructed part of the pancreas, there is uniform, diffuse atrophy and fibrosis of the acinar parenchyma. Calculi and intraductal protein plugs are uncommon.

Unlike acute pancreatitis, in chronic pancreatitis the morphologic changes in the pancreas are irreversible and often progressive, even if the cause (eg, alcoholism) is removed. This usually leads to permanent functional impairment as more and more acinar and islet cell mass is destroyed. The only exception is obstructive chronic pancreatitis, in which there may be improvement both morphologically and functionally when the obstruction is relieved.

The terms "recurrent acute" and "recurrent or relapsing chronic pancreatitis" are no longer used. They referred to repetitive episodes of pancreatic inflammation in patients with either of the two forms of the disease.

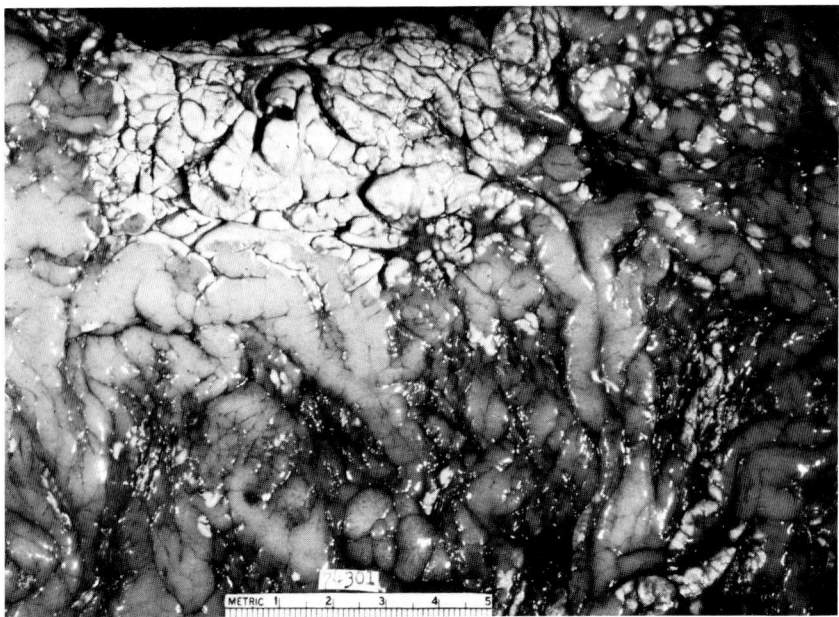

FIGURE 2.1. Acute pancreatitis. Peripancreatic fat with confluent chalky white patches of fat necrosis is shown (top). (Courtesy of EC Klatt, MD)

PATHOLOGY OF ACUTE PANCREATITIS

According to the Marseille definition, acute pancreatitis exhibits a spectrum of lesions, ranging from mild to severe.[3] These two forms grade into each other, and sharp separation is not always possible.

Mild Form

The mild form of acute pancreatitis is characterized by peripancreatic fat necrosis and interstitial edema of the pancreas. This results in a pale, boggy pancreas that may be diffusely enlarged. It is characterized by the collection of fluid between the pancreatic lobules. This fluid contains varying numbers of neutrophils depending on the severity of the process. The parenchymal architecture of the pancreas is preserved however, and there is little or no acinar necrosis. Fat necrosis presents grossly as pathognomonic, discrete, white or pale yellow, opaque, lusterless patches in the peripancreatic fat, omentum, and mesentery (Fig. 2.1). The patches of fat necrosis consist microscopically of clusters of dead fat cells with ghostlike outlines that are first pale pink and then become basophilic when the released free fatty acid combines with calcium to form soaps.

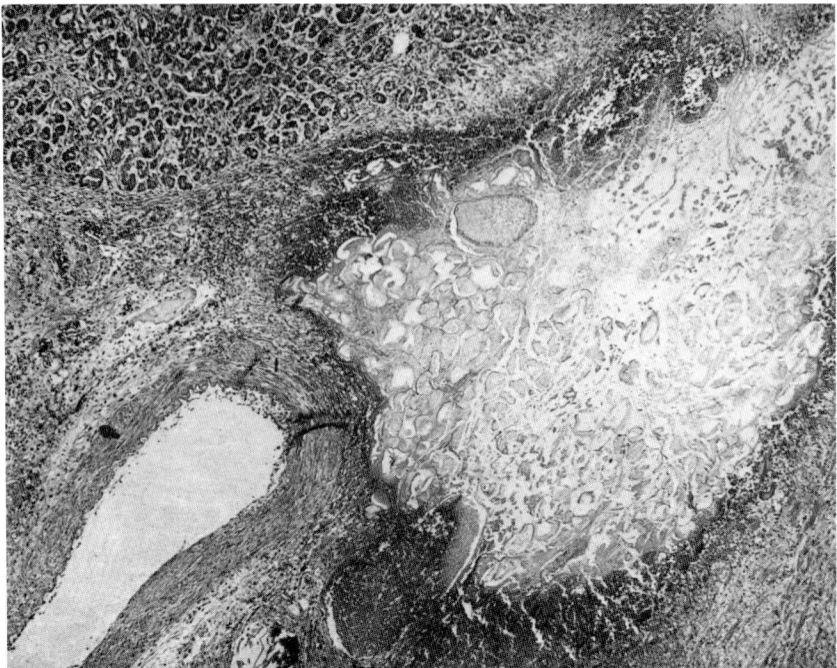

FIGURE 2.2. Acute pancreatitis. Fat necrosis (right) surrounded by advancing zone of inflammation is shown, extending into the pancreatic parenchyma (top) and an artery (left) (× 50). Courtesy of EC Klatt, MD)

Severe Form

In the severe form of acute pancreatitis, fat necrosis is more extensive and interstitial fat in the pancreas is involved. The free fatty acids released from the fat cells are intensely irritating,[4] and cause patchy necrosis of pancreatic acinar cells and blood vessels, with hemorrhage and thrombosis. The result is an enlarged, firm pancreas with patches of fat necrosis, covered with reddish-black clotted blood. Blood-stained fluid is present in the lesser sac. The necrotic tissue may become liquified, leaving a collection of semisolid, formless, dark material.

Severe acute pancreatitis appears microscopically as a mixture of necrosis, inflammation, and hemorrhage. Necrosis of fat is prominent; the pale staining areas of dead fat are surrounded by a zone of suppuration, with infiltration of neutrophils (Fig. 2.2). Acinar lumens may become dilated and the height of acinar cells diminished, leading to formation of ductlike structures known as tubular complexes. The glandular parenchyma also is involved by necrosis that first affects the periphery of the lobules, with leukocytic exudate adjacent. Necrosis of blood vessels leads to hemorrhage, and extravasation of the blood may permeate the entire interstitium, resulting in a swollen, dark reddish-black gland. Areas of relatively uninvolved parenchyma may persist, forming residual yellowish islands. Single or multiple abscesses may form around the necrotic tissue, with or without secondary infection.[5] Such abscesses often are multilocular, and they tend to burrow into the retroperitoneal tissues. Another complication is pancreatic pseudocyst, a collection of fluid adjacent to the pancreas contained within a wall of inflamed fibrous tissue.[5]

Ultrastructural Changes in Acute Pancreatitis

Electron microscopy reveals that acute pancreatitis is characterized by loss of zymogen granules. According to Willemer and Adler, the tubular complexes are degenerating acinar cells that have lost their secretory and membrane characteristics.[6] Other changes include disintegration of acinar cells, accumulation of platelets and leukocytes in vascular lumens, alterations in basal lamina, and extravasation of blood with deposition of fibrin.[7]

1. Sarles H, ed. *Pancreatitis: Symposium of Marseille, 1963*. Basel: S Karger; 1965.
2. Sarner M, Cotton PB. Classification of pancreatitis. *Gut* 1984;25:756–759.
3. Singer M, Gyr K, Sarles H. Revised classification of pancreatitis: report of the Second International Symposium on the Classification of Pancreatitis in Marseille, France, March 28–30, 1984. *Gastroenterology* 1985;89:683–690.
4. Schmitz-Moorman P. Comparative radiological and morphological study of the human pancreas. *Pathol Res Pract* 1981;171:325–355.
5. Cruickshank AH. *Pathology of the Pancreas*. New York: Springer-Verlag; 1986.
6. Willemer S, Adler G. Histochemical and ultrastructural characteristics of tubular complexes in human acute pancreatitis. *Dig Dis Sci* 1989;34:46–55.
7. Bockman DE, Buchler M, Beger HG. Ultrastructure of human acute pancreatitis. *Int J Pancreatol* 1986;1:141–153.

Chapter 3

Pathogenic Mechanisms of Pancreatitis

JORGE E. VALENZUELA
ANDRÉ RIBET

In 1986 Chiari proposed that digestive enzymes were involved in the pathogenesis of acute pancreatitis and that pancreatitis resulted from "autodigestion."[1] Thus proteolytic enzymes and lipases were considered responsible for the local inflammation, necrosis, and hemorrhage. When liberated into the circulation, they produced multiple organ alterations often observed in the disease. In patients with acute pancreatitis, both active proteolytic enzymes and phospholipase A_2 have been detected in pancreatic tissue and free proteases have been identified in pancreatic juice.

TRYPSIN

Trypsin is probably important in initiating the cascade of events in pancreatitis, since active trypsin infused into the pancreatic duct of dogs causes edema and hemorrhage. This probably represents a dual effect of the enzyme: it increases vascular permeability by releasing histamine and kallikrein, which converts kininogens to kinins and plasminogen to plasmin, and it can cause direct vascular damage and thrombosis, leading to tissue necrosis. This is observed after it is given as a subcutaneous injection. In addition to its direct effects, trypsin initiates the cascade of activation of other enzymes, including the release of active elastase, which aggravates vascular and cellular damage (Table 3.1).

Lipase has also been proposed to play a key role in the pathogenesis of pancreatic necrosis. Lipase hydrolyses triglycerides to produce fatty acids. These have a marked destructive effect on pancreatic cells by destroying the cell membranes. Hypertriglyceridemia is often associated with pancreatitis. It is possible that the resultant increased substrate causes lipase to generate a high local concentration of toxic breakdown products. Phospholipase A_2 has also received much attention since high concentrations of it are detected in necrotic pancreatic tissue of patients who died of acute pancreatitis. Moreover, high levels of this enzyme are found in the blood and

TABLE 3.1. Schematic Representation of the Possible Biochemical Events Initiating Pancreatitis and Causing Systemic Damage

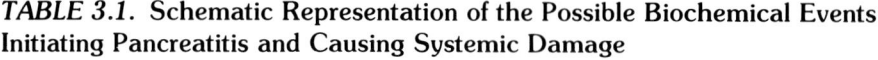

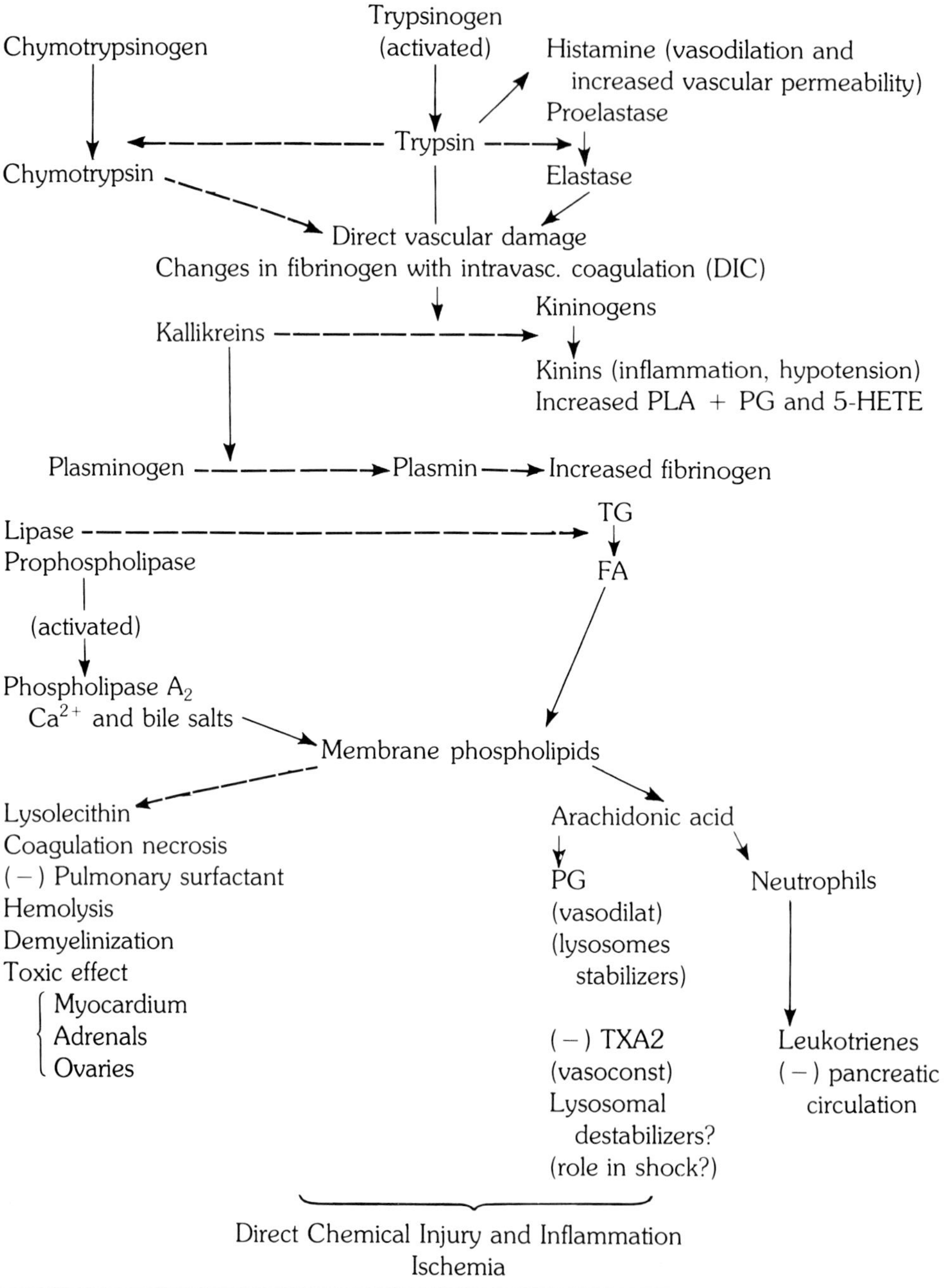

```
                              Trypsinogen
                              (activated)     Histamine (vasodilation and
   Chymotrypsinogen                ↘              increased vascular permeability)
            ↘                       ↗          Proelastase
             ↘         ←---------- Trypsin  ---→    ↓
   Chymotrypsin ↘                    ↓           Elastase
                  ↘                   ↓           ↙
                   → Direct vascular damage
            Changes in fibrinogen with intravasc. coagulation (DIC)
                                      ↓            Kininogens
              Kallikreins  ----------→              ↓
                    |                              Kinins (inflammation, hypotension)
                    |                              Increased PLA + PG and 5-HETE
                    ↓
   Plasminogen  ----------→ Plasmin ---→ Increased fibrinogen
                                                TG
   Lipase  -----------------------------→       ↓
   Prophospholipase                             FA
        |
     (activated)
        ↓
   Phospholipase A₂
   Ca²⁺ and bile salts  ↘
                          → Membrane phospholipids
   Lysolecithin ←                       ↓             ↘
   Coagulation necrosis                 Arachidonic acid
   (−) Pulmonary surfactant              ↓
   Hemolysis                            PG              Neutrophils
   Demyelinization                      (vasodilat)       |
   Toxic effect                         (lysosomes        |
     ⎧ Myocardium                        stabilizers)     |
     ⎨ Adrenals                                           ↓
     ⎩ Ovaries                          (−) TXA2        Leukotrienes
                                        (vasoconst)    (−) pancreatic
                                        Lysosomal         circulation
                                        destabilizers?
                                        (role in shock?)
                        ⎴⎴⎴⎴⎴⎴⎴⎴⎴⎴⎴⎴⎴⎴⎴⎴⎴⎴⎴⎴⎴⎴⎴⎴⎴⎴⎴⎴
                        Direct Chemical Injury and Inflammation
                                        Ischemia
```

(−) = decreased

TABLE 3.2. Possible Levels of Enzyme Activation

Intracellular
  Basolateral acinar cell "escape" or crinophagia: result from overstimulation with increased release of CCK?

Intrapancreatic Duct
  Spontaneous autoactivation of trypsin?
  Increased pancreatic duct permeability?

Increased Duodenopancreatic Reflux
  Increased biliary elimination of enterokinase?

---

the peritoneal fluid of patients with acute pancreatitis. Furthermore injection of phospholipase A_2 combined with bile salts into the pancreatic ducts of rats produces pancreatic damage, similar to that observed in humans. This probably results from the conversion of biliary lecithin to lysolecithin, which is highly toxic and may be responsible for coagulation necrosis, the breakdown of lipoproteins of both cell membranes and organelles, and the liberation of other toxic substances into the circulation.[2]

Direct release of phospholipase A_2 into circulation also appears to cause hemolysis and direct damage in distant organs. For instance, in the lungs it may cause pulmonary edema by altering the pulmonary surfactant level. In the central nervous system it may cause demyelinization, which may be responsible for the so-called pancreatic encephalopathy. Similar alterations probably occur in the myocardium, adrenals, and ovaries (see Table 3.1).

All the possible events triggered by trypsin activation or lipase release seem to converge into two main mechanisms of injury: direct chemical insult with inflammation, and ischemia. Under normal conditions there are at least four protective mechanisms to prevent proteases from becoming active. First, enzymes are synthesized as proenzymes, an inactive form. Second, they are stored in zymogen granules, separated from the cytoplasm by the zymogen granule membrane. Third, the internal milieu of zymogen granules and condensing vacuoles is acidic in nature, promoting the aggregation of proenzymes and preventing activation. Fourth, a trypsin inhibitor is secreted into the pancreatic juice.[3]

Nevertheless, for unknown reasons and under a wide variety of conditions, this activation appears to occur and pancreatitis develops. How could pancreatic enzyme activation take place?

Premature protease activation could occur hypothetically at three different levels (Table 3.2).

Intracellular Activation

Intracellular activation would occur if trypsin escaped from the protective environment of the zymogen granule and found more adequate conditions for spontaneous activation or was activated by other elements within the cytoplasm. There is some evidence that during experimental pancreatitis induced in rats by infusion of supramaximal doses of cerulein, newly synthesized proteins (enzymes) are released into the cytoplasm and into the peripancreatic tissue through the basolateral membrane ("basolateral escape"). Increased release of cholecystokinin (CCK) with pancreatic overstimulation has never been demonstrated clinically, however. Thus, the relevance of this model to human disease is unclear. In another model of experimental pancreatitis in young female mice fed a choline-deficient diet supplemented by ethionine, an admixture of zymogen granules and lysosomal contents seems to take place (crinophagia). Under these conditions activation of trypsinogen by one of the lysosomal hydrolases (cathepsin B) could take place.[4] Although there is no direct evidence that the pH of the zymogen granule may be altered during pancreatitis, some observations suggest that chronic alcohol intake may alter the intracellular vesicle acidification mechanism.

Another possibility could be activation of trypsinogen by plasmin or thrombin. Several conditions associated with pancreatitis (eg, ischemia, anoxia, sepsis) could increase the formation of plasminogen with release of plasmin; this can activate trypsin. Based on pathologic data, there is evidence that this process would occur more likely in the periphery of the acinar cells. It is not clear, however, how the proteases are exposed to the plasmin. Additional studies are needed to clarify this last hypothesis.

Intrapancreatic Duct Activation of Trypsin and Reflux to the Parenchyma

There is some evidence for the presence of active trypsin in the pancreatic juice of patients with chronic calcified alcoholic pancreatitis. This could occur by autoactivation of trypsinogen, but knowledge of the conditions within pancreatic juice do not favor this possibility. In fact, studies showed that when a small amount of active trypsin was added to pancreatic juice, it was rapidly degraded. In addition, the enzyme "Y" present in pancreatic juice degrades trypsinogen rapidly and seems to constitute an additional protective mechanism for the prevention of autoactivation.[3]

There is some evidence that pancreatic duct permeability can be altered. Several studies have demonstrated that an increase of duct permeability may allow back-diffusion of enzymes into the interstitium and blood. If the enzymes are active, pancreatitis could develop. For instance, acute edematous pancreatitis can be induced in cats by perfusing activated pancreatic enzymes through the pancreatic ducts after pretreatment with oral ethanol or intraductal bile.[5] This mechanism could explain biliary tract-related and alcohol-related pancreatitis. Nevertheless, there is no direct evidence for this mechanism in the human disease.

Increased Duodenopancreatic Reflux

According to the increased duodenopancreatic reflux hypothesis, pancreatic juice reaches the intestine, where trypsinogen is activated by enterokinase. There it mixes with bile and other components of duodenal content (eg, bacteria), and refluxes through the sphincter of Oddi, into the pancreatic ducts. This hypothesis is supported by observations on experimental hemorrhagic pancreatitis associated with a duodenal blind loop in dogs. The clinical counterpart for this condition is that of pancreatitis associated with duodenal loop obstruction. In patients who have had sphincterotomy or sphincteroplasty, however, where free reflux occurs frequently, pancreatitis is not observed.

Pancreatitis that occurs after endoscopic retrograde pancreatography (ERP) is an example of pancreatitis caused by pancreatic duct "reflux." It should be noted, however, that pancreatitis after ERP is relatively rare (less than 1%) and is more likely to occur when excessive pressure to inject the contrast material is used.

A different alternative based on the enterohepatic circulation of enterokinase has been proposed. There is evidence that enterokinase can enter portal blood and is cleared normally into the bile by the hepatocytes. In the presence of an alcoholic fatty liver, however, the enterokinase concentration in the bile increases. If regurgitation of bile into the pancreatic ductal system occurred, this could lead to intraductal activation of proteases. There is also some evidence that enterokinase may increase in the bile of postoperative patients, this suggests that peak increments of bile enterokinase could occur under certain circumstances.[6]

CLINICAL CONDITIONS ASSOCIATED WITH PANCREATITIS

Gallstones and alcoholism are the two most common conditions associated with pancreatitis. Together they account for about 75% of cases of pancreatitis. There is consensus that biliary stones may cause acute pancreatitis, whereas chronic alcohol ingestion is more frequently related to chronic pancreatitis. Acute episodes of pancreatitis in alcoholics occur most of the time when there is some chronic damage already established.

A long list of conditions is associated with acute and chronic pancreatitis (Table 3.3), and the mechanisms in most of these conditions remain unknown. "Idiopathic" pancreatitis still represents the third most common form, accounting for approximately 20% of all acute cases.

Pancreatitis Associated with Biliary Tract Disease

Several epidemiologic studies confirm that biliary stones are one of the most common factors associated with acute pancreatitis. The variable rates (40% to 70%) are determined by the different incidence of gallstones in various areas of the world.

Early in this century Opie described an autopsy case of hemorrhagic pancreatitis with a gallstone impacted in the ampulla of Vater. He proposed that the normal flow of bile into the duodenum was prevented by the stone.[7] Instead bile refluxed into the pancreatic duct through a short common channel that connected the two ducts just proximal to the stone. This caused pancreatitis. Claude Bernard should be given credit for suspecting the association between bile and pancreatitis, since he had produced experimental pancreatitis in dogs earlier by injecting bile and olive oil into the pancreatic ducts.[8] Since that time numerous experiments have confirmed that injec-

TABLE 3.3. Conditions Associated with Pancreatitis

Acute	Chronic
Biliary tract disease	Chronic alcoholism
Chronic alcoholism	Obstruction of the pancreatic duct
Obstruction of the pancreatic duct	Tropical (malnutritional)
Ischemia	Cystic fibrosis
Drugs	Hereditary
Infectious agents	Shwachman's syndrome
Postoperative	Enterokinase deficiency
Trauma	Isolated pancreatic enzyme deficiencies
Post ERCP	Idiopathic
Metabolic diseases	
After renal transplant	
Scorpion venom poisoning	
Penetrating peptic ulcer	
Hereditary	
Miscellaneous	
Idiopathic	

tion of bile into the pancreatic ducts may cause pancreatitis and it was proposed that the mechanism involved bile activation of trypsinogen. There are several objections to this interpretation, however. First, the pressure applied in the experimental situation usually exceeded that found under physiologic conditions. Therefore the pancreatitis might be caused by physical ductal disruption rather than enzymatic digestion. Although it has been shown that bile can induce necrosis, this occurs without evidence that it activates trypsinogen. An impacted stone with a common channel that would favor bile reflux to the pancreatic duct is not always found in biliary pancreatitis; however, transient obstruction of the biliary and pancreatic duct does appear to take place in patients with gallstone pancreatitis. Almost 90% of these patients had gallstones in their feces after an acute attack, suggesting an etiologic connection between the passage of the stones into the duodenum and the onset of the pancreatitis. Urgent endoscopic investigation of patients with gallstone pancreatitis demonstrated the presence of impacted stones in the ampulla. The clinical improvement that occurs after removal of these stones adds further support to the obstruction proposal.[9]

It is possible that other mechanisms induced by common bile duct obstruction could participate in the pathogenesis of gallstone pancreatitis. For instance, there is evidence that increased bile acid concentration in the blood increases pancreatic flow rate. The mechanism of this effect is unclear, although an increment in plasma levels of secretin occurs when bile acid concentration in the blood is increased.

Alcoholic Pancreatitis

Most alcoholics with pancreatitis have morphologic changes suggestive of chronic damage to the gland. In autopsy studies of chronic alcoholics whose death was attributed to acute pancreatitis, however, more than half of them had no conclusive histologic evidence of chronic pancreatitis.[10] In a group of alcoholics with acute pancreatitis, functional evaluation did not reveal exocrine insufficiency. The pathogenic mechanisms of this acute alcoholic pancreatitis remains unknown (11–13).

Three current hypotheses of the pathogenesis of alcoholic pancreatitis exist.

Direct Metabolic Effect

The direct metabolic effect hypothesis postulates that pancreatic damage results from a direct cytotoxic effect of alcohol on acinar cells. There is some evidence that pancreatic damage may result from pancreatic ethanol oxidation. Although the total amount of extrahepatic alcohol dehydrogenase (ADH) is about one tenth that found in the liver, there is evidence that ethanol is metabolized in the pancreas. Ethanol uptake by the pancreatic cells takes place by simple diffusion and is proportional to blood levels of alcohol. When the latter reaches 25 mM, ethanol concentration in the pancreatic cells is near the Vmax of pancreatic ADH.[14] This results in increased production of intermediate alcohol metabolites like acetate that may be partially used for lipid biosynthesis. It has been observed that ethanol stimulates incorporation of carbon 14-labeled acetate into pancreatic lipids during the course of acute and chronic intoxication. This appears to be the mechanism by which ethanol stimulates lipogenesis.

In addition, the pancreas requires large amounts of energy to perform its functions of protein synthesis and secretion. In fact, it has been demonstrated that 9 times more fatty acid is oxidized by the pancreas than by the liver and that oxidation of fatty acids and glucose constitute comparable sources of energy for the pancreas. Finally, there is evidence that although ethanol decreases pancreatic oxidation of acetate and fatty acids, it provides at the same time a low source of energy.[15]

In summary, ethanol oxidation by the pancreas decreases the energy generated by fatty acids and glucose oxidation. At the same time it stimulates biosynthesis of pancreatic lipids, a process that consumes energy. These biochemical observations provide the basis for understanding the ultrastructural changes observed in pancreatic tissue from chronic alcoholic patients. These reveal fat accumulation in the acinar cells with changes similar to those observed in the hepatocytes of alcoholics.[16] It is not known how these chronic changes could lead to acute pancreatitis, however. It is possible that the pancreas of chronic alcoholics affected by the metabolic changes described was more susceptible to events that normally would not produce pancreatitis. Among these factors could be ischemia, excessive secretory stimulation after a large meal (excessive release of CCK?), increased plasma free fatty acid concentration, or other unknown factors. These factors, acting by unknown mechanisms, could precipitate bouts of acute pancreatitis in chronic alcoholic patients without chronic pancreatitis.

Protein Plug Hypothesis

About half of alcoholic patients have well-established chronic morphologic and functional changes in the pancreas when they have the first clinical evidence of acute pancreatitis. Morphologically, besides the sclerosis with destruction of the parenchyma, there is a variable degree of dilation of segments of the duct system. Most often these dilations are related to strictures, intraductal protein plugs, and calculi. The following sequence of events seem to take place.

Chronic alcohol ingestion in experimental animals and human subjects causes changes in the character of pancreatic secretion. There is enhanced secretion of protein and impaired water and bicarbonate secretion, resulting in an hyperconcentrated juice. Studies on pure pancreatic secretion from chronic alcoholics also have revealed changes in the trypsin–trypsin inhibitor ratio as well as increased secretion of lysosomal enzymes.[17] Furthermore, it has been observed that other proteins are increased (eg, lactoferrin, albumin, and globulins). These last two proteins probably reflect increased permeability of the pancreatic duct barrier.

Another metabolic factor affecting the flow of pancreatic secretion in alcoholics is that increased levels of acetate in the blood and in the pancreas inhibit pancreatic secretion of water. This lowers the pH of the pancreatic juice.[14] All these changes could favor precipitation of proteins in the pancreatic ducts and eventual formation of stones. Sarles has provided additional information regarding the formation of calculi in these patients.[11] He proposes that protein plugs and calculi represent different stages of pancreatic lithogenesis and that the pancreatic stone protein (PSP), a stabilizer present in normal pancreatic juice, is decreased in patients with chronic alcoholic pancreatitis. Evidence for decreased PSP in chronic alcoholics before they develop pancreatitis has not been reported but pure pancreatic juice of patients with calcified pancreatitis of different causes was found to contain lower levels of PSP. Furthermore, the PSP gene expression is lower in these patients.[18]

Increased Pancreatic Duct Permeability Hypothesis

The increased pancreatic duct permeability hypothesis is based on observations on experimental models of acute pancreatitis after retrograde injection of duodenal juice into the pancreatic ducts. When these experiments are done on alcohol intoxicated rats, more pancreatic damage is observed compared with control rats. An analogy with the gastric mucosal barrier was postulated by Reber et al.[19] after observations that the cat pancreatic duct was relatively impermeable to molecules larger than 3000 d. Alcohol administered intragastrically increased pancreatic duct permeability. This allowed leakage of enzymes into the interstitium, with subsequent acute inflammatory changes.

In conclusion, the pathophysiology of alcoholic pancreatitis is not clear. Although chronic calcified pancreatitis may be explained by the protein plug hypothesis, the mechanism of acute pancreatitis in chronic alcoholics without the obvious morphologic changes of chronic pancreatitis remains uncertain. The influence of nutritional and genetic factors deserve further investigation (Table 3.4).

Pancreatitis Caused by Obstruction of the Pancreatic Duct

Several anatomic conditions cause pancreatitis by obstructing the pancreatic duct:

TABLE 3.4. **Pathogenesis of Alcoholic Pancreatitis**

Chronic Alcoholism
(Malnutrition, Genetic Factors, Smoking?)

With chronic pancreatitis	Without chronic pancreatitis
	Precipitating factors
Obstruction	Back diffusion?
(caused by)	Ischemia?
Protein plugs	Increased CCK release?
(as a result of)	Increased free FA?
Decreased PSP secretion	Increased fat content in acinar cells?
Changes in protein secretion,	Increased ethanol oxidation?
blood acetate levels	Increased synthesis of lipids?

1. Pancreatic cancer or ampullary carcinoma can cause pancreatitis in the portion of the gland distal to the obstruction. This has been found in up to 10% of cases of pancreatic cancer, and in some instances the episode of acute pancreatitis led to the diagnosis of pancreatic cancer.

2. Pancreas divisum is a congenital anomaly of the pancreatic duct system with failure of the ducts of the ventral and dorsal pancreas to fuse. It seems to occur in 5% to 7% of the general population. In most instances these persons are free of symptoms. Several reports, however, have attributed episodes of acute pancreatitis to pancreas divisum. In these patients there is presumed to be a relative stenosis of the accessory papilla that has become the major outflow tract for pancreatic secretion. Convincing dilation of the dorsal duct with a normal ventral duct rarely occurs, however. A provocative test with dilation of the dorsal pancreatic duct after secretin injection has been proposed,[20] but similar dilation has been observed in healthy subjects. The diagnosis of pancreas divisum is made by endoscopic pancreatography. More recent studies of the accessory papilla suggest that it contains a true sphincter. Manometric studies of the papilla are technically difficult, especially in patients with a narrowed papilla, and are of questionable practical value. It is now generally accepted that in most cases of pancreatitis the finding of pancreas divisum is coincidental. In a few cases pancreas divisum may be responsible for the pancreatitis, but it is not possible to reliably distinguish between the two in most instances.[21]

3. Parasitic infestations. Migration of parasites like *Ascaris lumbricoides* and *Clonorchis sinensis* (more common in Asians with clinical symptoms of cholangitis) into the pancreatic ducts may cause pancreatitis by obstruction of the lumen.

4. Duodenal diverticula. Juxtaduodenal diverticula are detected by upper gastrointestinal barium examination in about 6% of subjects, who in most instances are asymptomatic. There is a higher incidence of gallstones and pancreatitis in these patients, however. The gallstones are primarily pigmented stones, suggesting that obstruction and infection play a pathogenic role in their formation. It is not known whether pancreatitis results from the associated biliary stones or whether the diverticula cause obstruction of the pancreatic duct.

5. Rare cases of pancreatitis have been described associated with choledochocele or common bile duct cyst. It has been proposed that extrinsic compression (obstruction) or bile regurgitation into the pancreatic duct could be involved.
6. In some patients with recurrent idiopathic pancreatitis, elevated sphincter of Oddi basal pressure and sphincter dysmotility have been observed. This suggests that a functional obstruction could be the cause of the pancreatitis.

Ischemia as a Factor in Pancreatitis

A relationship between ischemia and pancreatitis has been suspected for many years. The pancreas should be added to the list of organs that may suffer from hypoperfusion secondary to shock or hypovolemia. This suggestion is based on clinical, experimental, and histologic evidence. For instance, acute pancreatitis occurs in cases with vasculitis, such as polyarteritis nodosa, systemic lupus erythematosus, thrombotic thrombocytopenic purpura, Henoch-Schönlein purpura, and necrotizing angiitis secondary to drugs. It is associated with malignant hypertension, atheromatous emboli after cardiopulmonary bypass, and oligemic shock, especially when there is concomitant acute tubular necrosis.

Pancreatitis can be produced experimentally by arterial occlusion, venous ligation, or intravascular injection of microspheres. In the ex vivo isolated purfused canine pancreas, ischemia causes edema that suggests capillary injury. There is also evidence that the lesions may result in part from the ischemia–reperfusion process with generation of oxygen-derived free radicals. In addition, in the isolated perfused pancreas, hypoxia and ischemia release lysosomal enzymes and a myocardial depressant factor that may further aggravate hypovolemia.

Tissue from patients dying of necrotising pancreatitis or from those who died during surgery revealed that pancreatic necrosis was frequently found in the microcirculatory periphery of the pancreatic lobule when shock was a prominent part of the clinical picture. Microthrombi in the blood vessels, platelet accumulation within and surrounding the vessels, and fibrin deposits in the connective tissue were also described. Moreover, other autopsy studies revealed that a number of patients with pancreatitis in whom the diagnosis was not made during life had had frequent episodes of circulatory failure before death. This suggested that ischemia could have played a pathogenic role. Thus, the real incidence of pancreatitis related to ischemia may not be known and may have been underestimated.

Drug-Induced Pancreatitis

A relationship between the ingestion of a number of drugs and the occurrence of pancreatitis has been proposed in many reports. There is a remarkable lack of documentation and information about the pathogenesis and dose relationship, however. Mallory and Kern critically reviewed all the reported cases of pancreatitis related to drugs and concluded that only a few drugs had a definitive association with pancreatitis.[22]

Drugs Definitively Associated with Pancreatitis

AZATHIOPRINE

Clinical pancreatitis occurred in 6.2% of 116 patients who participated in the National Cooperative Crohn's Disease Study and received azathioprine alone compared with those who received placebo, prednisone, or sulfasalazine. These cases had received between 50 and 150 mg of azathioprine per day for 13 to 21 days before clinical evidence of pancreatitis was noted.[23]

This form of pancreatitis can also be observed after renal transplantation and during the course of treatment of chronic hepatitis. The mechanism for azathioprine-associated pancreatitis is attributed to hypersensitivity reaction.

6-MERCAPTOPURINE

This drug, a metabolite of azathioprine has also been used in the treatment of Crohn's disease. Pancreatitis was seen in 3.25% of 400 patients receiving 6-Mercaptopurine (6-MP). The dosage ranged from 50 to 100 mg daily and pancreatitis occurred within 8 to 32 days after the beginning of treatment. In a few cases, pancreatitis recurred when the patients were rechallenged with 6-MP. The mechanism of pancreatitis caused by azathioprine or 6-MP is unknown, although an allergic mechanism has been proposed.

DIURETICS

Chlorothiazide, hydrochlorothiazide, and furosemide have been related to pancreatitis. The frequency of pancreatitis caused by thiazides is not known, although up to 50% of a small group of patients receiving the drug had an increased serum amylase concentration. In general the severity of the symptoms increased with the dose and duration of the exposure. Seven fatalities have been reported and one autopsy study revealed inspissated intraductal secretions reminiscent of those described in the pancreas of chronic alcoholics. One experimental study observed that pancreatitis occurred in mice treated with chlorothiazide for 1 to 6 months.

ESTROGENS

There are many reports of pancreatitis in patients who received estrogens and a strong correlation was observed in relation to the concomitant elevation of the serum triglycerides level. Clinically pancreatitis seems to occur after at least 3 months of estrogen therapy and when serum triglycerides are markedly increased, usually above 3,500 mg/dL. It is not known how this elevated triglyceride level causes pancreatitis. Vascular thromboses were found in one autopsy study. There is no evidence that estrogens can cause pancreatitis independent of hypertriglyceridemia.

SULFONAMIDES

Although less frequent, the association between pancreatitis and ingestion of sulfonamides is convincing. When this occurs the symptoms of pancreatitis are often associated with fever, skin rash, and pruritus, suggesting an allergic mechanism. A recent observation that lymphocytes from a patient with sulfonamide-induced pancreatitis were stimulated in vitro by sulfa compounds appears to reinforce this hypothesis.

TETRACYCLINE

A direct relationship between the occurrence of pancreatitis, tetracycline dosage, and duration of the treatment has been noted. Almost invariably pancreatitis is accompanied by liver disease. It carries a serious prognosis, and in one series the mortality rate was more than 50%.

Other drugs definitely associated with pancreatitis are valproic acid and methyldopa.

Drugs Probably Associated with Pancreatitis

A probable association with pancreatitis was suggested after administration of L-asparaginase, chlorthalidone, corticosteroids, phenformin, and procainamide. The controversy regarding steroids is not over; although some authors have reported beneficial corticosteroid effect in the management of acute pancreatitis, one case report noted recurrence of pancreatitis when the patient was rechallenged with steroids.[24]

Drugs with No Convincing Evidence to Cause Pancreatitis

A large list of drugs has been proposed to cause pancreatitis but the evidence appears inadequate. This category included amphetamines, cholestyramine, cyproheptadine, propoxyphene, diazoxide, histamine, indomethacin, acetylsalicylic acid, isoniazid, opiates, rifampicin, acetaminophen, cimetidine, and metronidazole.

Infectious Agents

Pancreatitis seems to occur in a variety of systemic infections including *Mycoplasma pneumoniae,* mumps, Coxsackie viruses of group B, hepatitis, herpes simplex, infectious mononucleosis, and Legionnaire's disease. In some cases there are clinical manifestations including abdominal pain and tenderness with increase in serum amylase. The diagnosis is rarely made by surgical exploration. In most cases the association is suspected based on serologic evidence of increased antibody titers in patients with acute pancreatitis. In some patients with pancreatitis and increased mycoplasma pneumoniae titers, there was absence of respiratory symptoms.

Postoperative Pancreatitis

It is accepted that postoperative pancreatitis occurs more frequently after pancreatic, biliary, or gastric surgery, although it may occur in procedures remote from the pancreas. If the pancreas is incised, the risk of pancreatitis is greatly enhanced. Common bile duct exploration and sphincter manipulation are more frequently associated with postoperative pancreatitis. The incidence of pancreatitis seems to be higher when patients had a preoperative episode of pancreatitis. The clinical presentation is often severe and the pathogenesis is related to the mechanism of injury, for example, trauma, devascularization, or stricture.

Pancreatitis Secondary to Trauma

Trauma to the pancreas is estimated to occur in about 3% of penetrating injuries to the abdomen. A similar incidence is reported after abdominal blunt trauma. The pancreas can be damaged as a result of contusion, laceration, subcapsular hematomas, or rupture of the pancreatic duct system. Traumatic pancreatitis results from compression of the gland against the spine and the degree of inflammation is variable. This form of pancreatitis is observed after abdominal contusions received during a car accident when the steering wheel hits the periumbilical area, or in small children, after trauma to the abdomen caused by a bicycle handlebar. The clinical presentation may be severe and in some instances a fracture of the pancreatic duct with extravasation of contrast medium to the peritoneum may occur. This may explain the relatively high incidence of complications such as fistulas, abscesses, and pseudocysts that occur after traumatic pancreatitis.

Pancreatitis After Endoscopic Retrograde Cholangiopancreatography

It is relatively common (between 25 to 50% of procedures) to observe hyperamylasemia after endoscopic retrograde cholangiopancreatography (ERCP) but acute pancreatitis occurs more rarely (less than 1%). Excessive injection pressure appears to be the mechanism, since filling of the small pancreatic ducts is more often associated with pancreatitis. This complication of ERCP may be avoided by gentle pressure and the avoidance of overfilling of the duct system. The course is usually benign, although in some cases a pseudocyst, abscess, or death may follow.

Metabolic Diseases that Cause Pancreatitis

Hyperlipidemia

An association between hyperlipidemia and pancreatitis is suggested by several conditions. First, acute and recurrent pancreatitis occur in hyperlipidemia, specifically phenotypes I, IV, and V. Second, pancreatitis occurs more frequently in patients with congenital C-II apoprotein deficiency. Third, hypertriglyceridemia is frequently observed in alcohol-related and estrogen-related episodes of pancreatitis. Fourth, increased fasting serum triglycerides and impaired clearance of lipids after a fat load were observed in a group of patients after an acute episode of pancreatitis. This was true whether the attack was related to biliary tract disease or alcoholism; it was not associated with diabetes. Subsequent studies in this last group of patients suggest that they may have a preexisting lipid metabolism disorder.

The mechanism by which hypertriglyceridemia causes pancreatitis remains unknown. It has been suggested that lipase could increase the concentration of free fatty acids in the small vessels of the pancreas. Both triglycerides and fatty acids are toxic to the isolated perfused pancreas and pancreatitis induced by intraductal injection of bile and trypsin is more severe in animals fed a high-fat diet. The strong association between alcoholism, hyperlipidemia, and pancreatitis and the improvement of hyperlipidemia in some alcoholics that stop drinking raise the possibility that alcoholism and pancreatitis could in some cases cause hyperlipidemia.

Hyperparathyroidism

Although earlier studies suggested that pancreatitis was a relatively frequent complication of hyperparathyroidism, a review of over 1000 patients with primary hyperparathyroidism operated at the Mayo Clinic revealed that only 1.5% of them had a coexisting or previous history of pancreatitis.[25] This frequency does not differ significantly from that of other hospitalized patients. Most patients also had other factors such as gallstone or biliary tract disease that could be related to pancreatitis. Of further interest, cure of hyperparathyroidism in some cases did not affect the course of pancreatitis.[25] This study and the failure to induce pancreatitis in experimental hyperparathyroidism cast some doubt on the possible relationship between hyperparathyroidism and pancreatitis. Nevertheless, cases of pancreatitis related to hypercalcemia caused by other conditions such as multiple myeloma, metastatic cancer, sarcoidosis, and total parenteral nutrition have been described.

Pancreatitis After Renal Transplant

Definition of pancreatitis after renal transplant may be difficult since hyperamylasemia occurs frequently in patients with renal insufficiency. Acute pancreatitis has been reported in 2% to 6% of patients after renal transplantation. The pathogenic mechanism may be difficult to analyze since these patients are frequently taking immunosuppressive agents such as azathioprine and corticosteroids and they are exposed to opportunistic infections that may infect the pancreas. Some pancreatic injury may occur during left nephrectomy and splenectomy before transplantation. In some cases of pancreatitis after renal transplantation, pathologic examination of the pancreas has revealed some interstitial fibrosis, suggesting some form of chronic pancreatic damage. Histologic pancreatic abnormalities have been described in patients with chronic renal disease.

Pancreatitis After Scorpion Venom Poisoning

Cases of pancreatitis after a sting by the scorpion *Tityus trinitatis* have been reported from Trinidad. Some patients may have hyperamylasemia with no abdominal pain, although cases of hemorrhagic pancreatitis and death may occur, particularly in children.[26] The pathogenesis of this form of pancreatitis is unknown, but it is known from studies in dogs that the venom stimulates a secretion rich in enzymes (acetylcholine or CCK-like effect). In addition, the animals also developed edema of the papilla of Vater, suggesting that there may have been obstruction to the flow of secretion.

Pancreatitis Associated with Penetrating Peptic Ulcer

This is a situation more often cited than documented. It is conceivable that penetrating antral or duodenal ulcers could initiate some satellite inflammatory reaction in the adjacent gland, but it must occur rarely.

Hereditary Pancreatitis

This form of pancreatitis appears to be transmitted as an autosomal dominant trait. The pathogenesis remains unknown since these patients do not have a consistent metabolic or structural abnormality. Episodes of pancreatitis occur in these patients early in life (teens or early 20s) and generally have a good prognosis. It has not been determined whether a defect in secreting the pancreatic stone protein is present in patients with hereditary pancreatitis. There may be an increased likelihood for the development of pancreatic adenocarcinoma in these patients.

Tropical Pancreatitis (Malnutritional)

This form of pancreatitis occurs mainly in children and adolescents of developing countries where childhood malnutrition is common.[27] Tropical chronic pancreatitis is characterized by extensive pancreatic damage, fibrosis, and calcifications and is observed in countries such as Nigeria, Kerala (India), Indonesia, Thailand, Malawa, and Uganda. In contrast, in the pancreatic fibrosis observed in kwashiorkor, calcifications are rare, and this condition may improve after dietary balance has been restored. This has suggested that other factors could be involved in the pathogenesis of nutritional pancreatitis. A relationship between this form of pancreatitis and heavy consumption of cassava has been noted. It has been postulated that the presence of cyanhidric acid in the outer layers of the cassava root could have a direct toxic effect on the pancreas. The effect of cassava could also be indirect by depriving the pancreas of essential amino acids that are necessary for its functions. Other factors incriminated in this form of pancreatitis are zinc, copper, and selenium deficiencies. It has been postulated that chronic cyanide toxicity could be a common factor in the pathogenesis of malnutrition and in chronic alcoholic pancreatitis.[28]

Miscellaneous Causes of Pancreatitis

Cases of pancreatitis have been observed in a variety of other conditions, including anticholinesterase insecticide (organophosphate compounds) intoxication, during episodes of intermittent acute porphyria, chronic renal disease, afferent loop syndrome after Billroth II anastomosis, and fulminant hepatic failure. The pathogenesis of these cases is unclear. The observations are usually anecdotal and the relationship between the causative factor and the inflammation of the gland is not always firmly established.

References

1. Chiari H. Untitled. *Z. Heilk* 1896;17:69–96.
2. Nevalainen, TJ. The role of phospholipase A in acute pancreatitis. *Scand J Gastroenterol* 1980;15:641–650.
3. Rinderknecht H. Activation of pancreatic zymogens. *Dig Dis Sci* 1986;31:314–321.
4. Steer ML, Meldolesi JM. The cell biology of experimental pancreatitis. *N Engl J Med* 1987; 316:144–150.
5. Wedgwood KR, Farmer RC, Reber HA. A model of hemorrhagic pancreatitis in cats—role of 16, 16-dimethyl prostaglandin E2. *Gastroenterology* 1986;90:32–39.
6. Grant DAW, Talbot RW, Hermon-Taylor J. Catalytically active enterokinase in human bile. *Clin Chem Acta* 1984;142:39–45.
7. Opie EL. The etiology of acute hemorrhagic pancreatitis. *Bull Johns Hopkins Hosp* 1901; 12:182–190.
8. Bernard C. An Introduction to the Study of Experimental Medicine. Dover, New York, 1965.
9. Neptolemos JP, Carr-Locke DL, London NJ. Controlled trial of urgent endoscopic retrograde cholangiopancreatography and endoscopic sphincterotomy versus conservative treatment for acute pancreatitis due to gallstones. *Lancet* 1988;2:979–983.
10. Renner IG, Savage WT, Pantoja JL. Death due to acute pancreatitis: a retrospective analysis of 405 autopsy cases. *Dig Dis Sci* 1985;30:1005–1018.
11. Sarles H. Etiopathogenesis and definition of chronic pancreatitis. *Dig Dis Sci* 1986; 31:91S–107S.
12. Malagelada JR. The pathophysiology of alcoholic pancreatitis. *Pancreas* 1986;1:270–278.
13. Tiscornia OM, Dreiling DA. Physiospathogenic hypothesis of alcoholic pancreatitis: supranormal ecbolic stimulation of the "pancreon" units secondary to the loss of the negative component of pancreas innervation. *Pancreas* 1987;2:604–612.
14. Estival A, Clemente F, Ribet A. Ethanol metabolism by the rat pancreas during a chronic ethanol intoxication. *Toxicol Appl Pharmacol* 1981;61:155–165.
15. Calaeron-Attas P, Furnelle J, Christophe J. In vitro effects of ethanol and ethanol metabolism in the rat pancreas. *Biochim Biophys Acta* 1980;620:387–399.
16. Noronha M, Saldigano A, Ferreira-De-Almeida MJ, et al. Alcohol and the pancreas. Clinical associations and histopathology of animal pancreatic inflammation. *Am J Gastroenterol* 1981;76:114–119.
17. Renner IG, Rinderknecht H, Valenzuela JE, et al. Studies of pure pancreatic secretions in chronic alcoholic subjects without pancreatic insufficiency. *Scand J Gastroenterol* 1980; 15:241–244.
18. Multigner L, Sarles H, Lombardo D. Pancreatic Stone Protein II: implication in stone formation during the course of chronic calcifying pancreatitis. *Gastroenterology* 1985; 89:387–391.

19. Reber HA, Roberts C, Way LW. The pancreatic duct mucosal barrier. *Am J Surg* 1979; 137:128–134.
20. Warshaw AL, Simoene J, Shapiro RH, et al. Objective evaluation of ampullary stenoses with ultrasound and pancreatic stimulation. *Am J Surg* 1985;149:65–72.
21. Cotton PB. Pancreas Divisium. *Pancreas* 1988;3:245–247.
22. Mallory A, Kern F. Drug-induced pancreatitis: a critical review. *Gastroenterology* 1980; 78:813–820.
23. Sturdevant RA, Singleton JW, Julius JD, et al. Azathioprine-related pancreatitis in patients with Crohn's disease. *Gastroenterology* 1979;77:883–886.
24. Levine RA, McGuire RF. Corticosteroid-induced pancreatitis: a case report demonstrating recurrence with rechallenge. *Am J Gastroenterol* 1988;83:1161–1164.
25. Bess MA, Edis AJ, van Heerdon JA. Hyperparathyroidism and pancreatitis: chance or a causal association? *JAMA* 1980;243:246–247.
26. Bartholomew C. Acute scorpion pancreatitis in Trinidad. *Br Med J* 1970;1:666–668.
27. Pitchumoni CS. Pancreas in primary malnutrition disorders. *Am J Clin Nutr* 1973; 26:374–379.
28. Pitchumoni CS, Jain NK, Lowenfels AB. Chronic cyanide poisoning: unifying concept for alcoholic and tropical pancreatitis. *Pancreas* 1988;3:220–222.

Chapter 4

Clinical Presentation of Acute Pancreatitis

HOWARD A. REBER
JORGE E. VALENZUELA
HARTLEY COHEN

The typical attack of acute pancreatitis begins with severe and persistent epigastric or upper abdominal pain that radiates through to the back. It often follows the ingestion of a large meal and is associated with nausea and persistent vomiting and retching. The findings are the same regardless of the cause, even if the event represents an episode of acute pancreatic inflammation in a patient with chronic pancreatitis.

The pain may be more or less severe depending on the severity of the pancreatitis (eg, mild edematous versus severe hemorrhagic forms). Examination of the abdomen reveals tenderness most marked in the epigastrium, but sometimes present throughout. The bowel sounds are decreased or absent and peritoneal signs are rarely present initially. Usually there are no masses palpable; when one is present, it most often represents a swollen pancreas (phlegmon), pseudocyst, or abscess. The temperature is only mildly elevated (100 to 101°F, 38 to 38.5°C) in uncomplicated cases. There may be evidence of a pleural effusion, especially on the left side.

When the disease is more extensive, the patient may also exhibit evidence of profound fluid losses from sequestration of edema fluid or blood in the peripancreatic retroperitoneal spaces or in the peritoneal cavity (ascites). Then there may be severe dehydration, tachycardia, and hypotension. In about 1% of cases, a bluish color is evident around the umbilicus (Cullen's sign) or in the flanks (Grey Turner's sign) (Fig. 4.1). This represents blood that has dissected to those areas from the retroperitoneum around the pancreas in patients with hemorrhagic pancreatitis. Although the clinical presentation is often highly suggestive of the correct diagnosis, and the laboratory findings usually confirm it, it is important to stress that acute pancreatitis is a diagnosis of exclusion. Other acute upper abdominal conditions (perforated peptic ulcer, acute cholecystitis) must be considered in every case. An abrupt onset with boardlike abdomen is more commonly found with a perforated viscus (ie, perforated peptic ulcer). If doubt remains a laparotomy may be indicated for diagnosis, since the diseases with which acute pancreatitis are most likely to be confused are often lethal if not treated surgically.

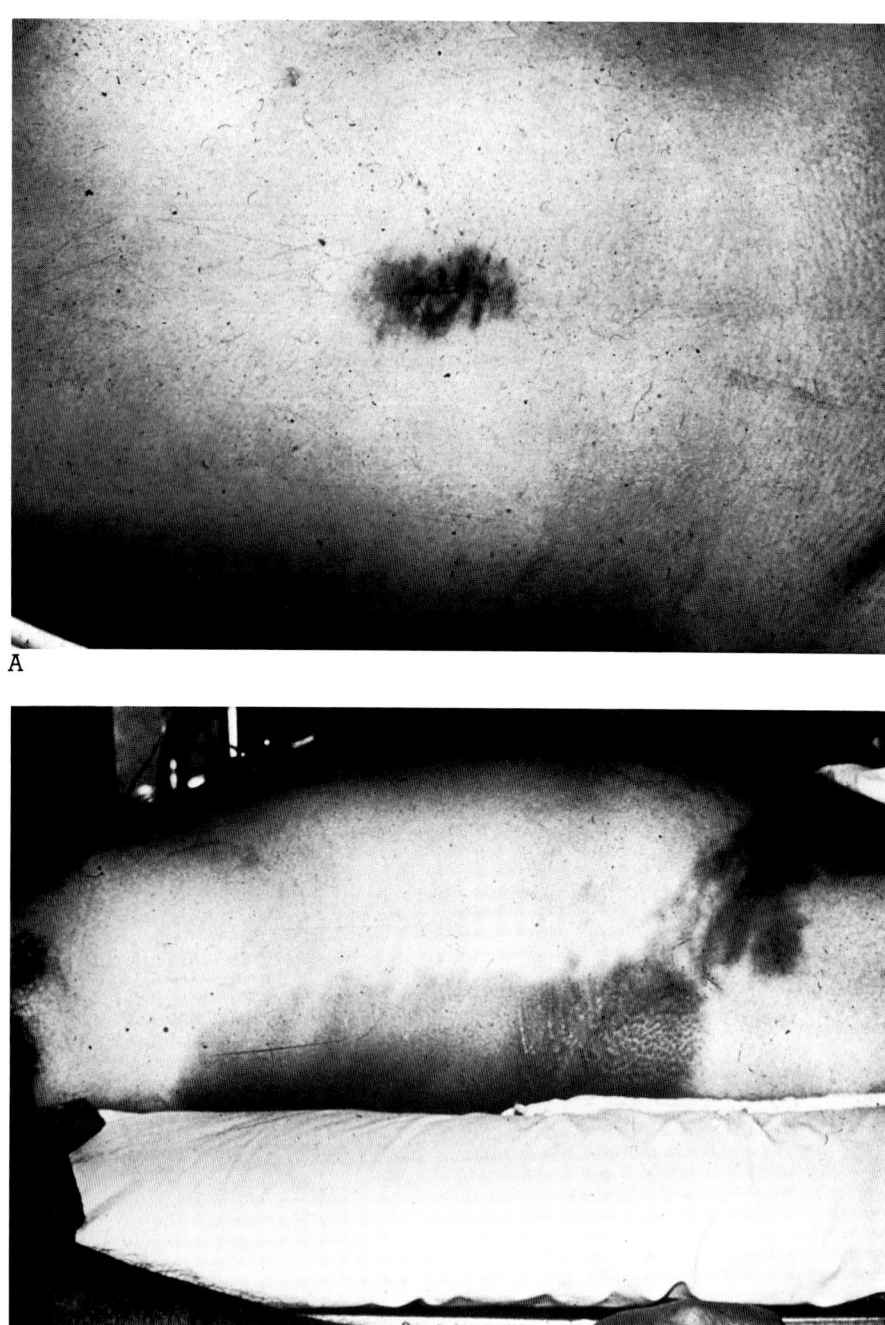

FIGURE 4.1. A: Ecchymoses around the umbilical area, Cullen's sign. B: Ecchymosis in the flank, Grey Turner's sign in a patient with severe hemorrhagic pancreatitis.

CLINICAL PRESENTATION

LABORATORY DIAGNOSIS OF ACUTE PANCREATITIS

The diagnosis of acute pancreatitis is made difficult by the lack of specific symptoms, and because laparotomy is rarely performed and histologic confirmation is unusual. In most cases of mild to moderate severity where spontaneous resolution occurs, the diagnosis may remain unproven. For these reasons, laboratory and imaging abnormalities are of paramount importance.

Biochemical alterations such as increased serum alanine-amino transferase and alkaline phosphatase, hyperbilirubinemia, and hematologic abnormalities like leukocytosis are nonspecific and occur in many abdominal emergencies. According to one study, however, elevation of serum glutamic-oxaloacetic transaminase (SGOT) suggested biliary pancreatitis.[1] Others have found that increased serum glutamic-pyruvic transaminase (SGPT) with an SGOT to SGPT ratio less than 1 also should raise the suspicion of biliary pancreatitis.[2]

Determinations of serum pancreatic enzymes have become the most widely accepted tests to support the diagnosis of acute pancreatitis.

Serum Amylase Concentration

Most of the amylase secreted by the pancreatic acinar cells reaches the duodenum. A small amount enters the blood, however, where it can be detected at levels usually less than 160 IU/dL. Other sources of amylase in the serum in addition to the pancreas include the salivary glands (isoamylase-S), with lesser contributions from the lungs and Fallopian tubes. Electrophoretic separation of the isoamylases reveals that about 40% of normal serum amylase is pancreatic in origin. A number of conditions affecting other organs without evidence of pancreatitis can cause hyperamylasemia and consequently decrease its specificity (Table 4.1). Although identification of pancreatic type (P) isoamylase can be done by electrophoresis, this is cumbersome and impractical for clinical use.

Although elevations of serum amylase concentration can occur in the absence of pancreatic inflammation, there are a number of examples where pancreatitis may be accompanied by normal amylase levels. For example, in one study of alcoholic patients with abdominal pain, nausea or vomiting, and ultrasonographic and CT changes compatible with pancreatitis, 32% of cases showed no elevations of serum amylase.[3] When pancreatitis occurs with hypertriglyceridemia with lactescent serum, elevated amylase concentration may not be detected until the serum is diluted. The factor that inhibits serum amylase remains unknown.

In spite of these limitations, serum amylase, if it is increased 3 or more times the upper limit of normal, has a specificity (normal values in cases without the disease) close to 100% and continues to be widely used as a first assay to diagnose acute pancreatitis. According to one study[4] hyperamylasemia has a sensitivity (abnormal values among all patients with acute pancreatitis demonstrated by pancreas imaging or laparotomy) of about 95%.

TABLE 4.1. **Causes of Hyperamylasemia (Other than Pancreatitis)**

Nonpancreatic: is predominantly salivary (S) isoamylase
  Salivary glands: Trauma, inflammation, ductal obstruction, radiation, chronic alcoholism
  Lungs: Tumors, pneumonia, tuberculosis
  Ovaries: Cysts, rupture ectopic pregnancy
  Prostate: Tumors
  Small bowel obstruction
  Diabetic ketoacidosis, cerebral trauma, thermal burns

Pancreatic: without pancreatitis is predominantly pancreatic (P) isoamylase
  Acute cholecystitis
  Perforated peptic ulcer
  Mesenteric infarction
  Renal failure
  Smoking (usually mild)
  Metastatic breast cancer
  Macroamylasemia (normal amylase bound to an abnormal serum protein which cannot be excreted by the kidney)
  Pancreatic duct obstruction (ie, ampullary tumors, post ERCP)
  After administration of secretin and cholecystokinin

Urinary Amylase Excretion

About 20% of the plasma amylase is filtered by the glomeruli. A large fraction is reabsorbed, whereas another is catabolized by the renal tubule. Amylase is cleared by the kidney with an amylase–creatinine clearance ratio (ACCR) of about 3%. During episodes of acute pancreatitis, urinary amylase excretion and the renal clearance of amylase are elevated because of the increased amount of enzyme that is filtered and its impaired tubular reabsorption. Because the creatinine clearance remains unchanged, the ACCR rises, often above 5%. Determination of urinary amylase excretion or ACCR adds little specificity to the diagnosis of pancreatitis, however, since they can both be elevated in other conditions, such as renal failure, after thoracic and cardiac surgery, in diabetic ketoacidosis, and after extensive burns. In summary, elevations of total serum amylase concentration, urinary amylase excretion, and ACCR are nonspecific and of limited value; specificity may be improved by determination of specific pancreatic isoamylase (P) levels; and normal serum P isoamylase levels may occur in acute pancreatitis and should not be the only criterion used to exclude the diagnosis.

Serum Lipase

The lack of specificity of amylase determinations prompted measurement of serum lipase to confirm the diagnosis of acute pancreatitis. Hyperlipasemia is more specific for pancreatitis since the pancreas is responsible for almost all of the lipase in the serum. Additional small amounts arise from sublingual secretion, the stomach, and the liver. The main disadvantage of serum lipase assay is methodologic. Serum lipase has been most commonly assayed by titrimetric, spectrophotometric, and turbidimetric methods that were based on the lipase capacity to liberate free fatty acids from an olive oil emulsion. The first titrimetric method (Cherry Crandall, 1932)[5] required a long period of incubation (16 to 24 hours) that limited its practical value. Current improved turbidimetric assays need between 30 minutes and 3 hours of incubation only and provide a more specific and sensitive measurement of lipase activity.

More recently a radioimmunoassay for human pancreatic lipase has become available (Nuclipase ^{125}I, Nuclin Diagnostics, Northbrook, IL). This assay measures the actual concentration of lipase instead of nonspecific lipolytic activity. Thus, it is less affected by the presence of high concentrations of other nonpancreatic lipases. Elevated serum lipase as determined by RIA seems to have a sensitivity and a specificity of about 90% and a high correlation with increments in serum pancreatic isoamylase.[6] An advantage of lipase measurement is that normal levels are detected in macroamylasemia and diabetic ketoacidosis. Hyperlipasemia may be observed in patients with renal insufficiency without evidence of pancreatic inflammation, acute cholecystitis, mesenteric infarction, perforated peptic ulcer and perforated intestine, obstructive jaundice, and fat embolism, however. Sequential measurement of pancreatic isoamylase and lipase in patients recovering from acute pancreatitis revealed that both enzymes remained elevated longer than total amylase.[7] Overall, serum lipase values above the upper limit of normal have a sensitivity and specificity of about 90%. In summary, assay of lipase is a reliable test and should be used more often in the diagnosis of pancreatitis. It seems to be as useful and more practical than the measurement of serum pancreatic isoamylase (P).

Trypsinogen

Because the pancreas appears to be the sole source of this proenzyme, determination of serum trypsinogen levels could have higher specificity for the diagnosis of acute pancreatitis.

Serum trypsinogen can be determined by two commercially available radioimmunoassay (RIA) kits (CIS Trypsik, Sorin Biomedica, Saluggia, Italy, and Behring Werke, Marburg, Germany). Many studies have reported increased levels of immunoreactive trypsinogen at the onset of acute pancreatitis. The diagnostic accuracy of this assay reveals that it is as sensitive and specific as measurement of pancreatic isoamylase.[7] Given the methodologic limitation of an RIA, however, the serum trypsinogen assay does not seem to offer advantages in simplicity and cost compared with measurement of pancreatic-isoamylase in the diagnosis of acute pancreatitis. Trypsinogen assay can distinguish between the hyperamylasemia caused by macroamylase and that caused by acute pancreatitis. Of greater interest, however, is that low serum levels below the lower limit of normal can be detected in about half of the patients with chronic pancreatitis. This has diagnostic value.

Elastase-1

Elastase-1 is produced exclusively by the pancreas, but the measurement of elastase-1 in the serum has been hampered by binding of this enzyme to serum inhibitors. An RIA has become commercially available (Elastase-1, Reakit, Abbott, Wiesbaden, Delkenheim, Germany). Different studies have reported that elastase-1 is consistently elevated in acute pancreatitis, with a sensitivity similar to that of pancreatic isoamylase. It is of interest that this enzyme has been found to be elevated in the serum several days after acute episodes of pancreatitis, whereas most other enzymes have returned to basal levels. Unfortunately elevated elastase-1 values are not specific since they can also be found in patients with chronic pancreatitis and pancreatic cancer. They also have been detected during the acute phase in patients with inflammatory bowel disease (IBD). It is not known whether this elevation of elastase-1 in IBD represents a true pancreatic inflammation, possibly caused by drugs used to treat IBD, or arises by another mechanism.

Miscellaneous Enzymes

There are diverse reports analyzing other enzymes or inhibitors in serum for the diagnosis of acute pancreatitis, including carboxypeptidase (enzymatic and RIA), acid ribonucleases (enzymatic), phospholipase A_2 (enzymatic), $\alpha_1$antitrypsin, trypsin inhibitor, and alpha-2-macroglubulin (radial immunodiffusion). To date none has proved useful.

Methemalbumin

Metheme (Hematin) is a breakdown product of hemoglobin that combines with albumin to form methemalbumin. In the hemorrhagic forms of pancreatitis, its concentration in the blood increases, inducing intravascular hemolysis. The appearance of methemalbumin in the blood is slow, however, and may take 72 hours or more. Most centers in the United States do not routinely perform this assay.

Assessment of Severity in Acute Pancreatitis

Acute pancreatitis is a self-limited condition in about 75% of cases. In the remaining 25% the course is severe, and death occurs in about one third of the cases. Early identification (within 48 hours of admission) of those patients at higher risk would allow more aggressive treatment for that subgroup. This would include transfer to an intensive care unit with continuous monitoring of central venous pressure, blood gases, renal function, assisted ventilation, and vigorous administration of fluids,

Algorithm for the Diagnosis of Acute Pancreatitis

Consider Pancreatitis in Patients with:
  Positive history of alcoholism or biliary stones or ingestion of estrogens, diuretics, steroids, azathioprine, hypercalcemia, hyperlipidemia, trauma.
  Negative history of peptic ulcer.

Who Complains of Midabdominal Pain:
  Radiating to the Back, Constant
  Frequently associated with nausea and vomiting and has on physical examination: Mild jaundice, tachycardia, hypotension.
   Abdominal tenderness.
   Bowel sounds may be decreased.

Laboratory Abnormalities Are:
  Leukocytosis, elevation of bilirubin, alkaline phosphatase, transaminases, LDH and hypocalcemia.
  Serum amylase and lipase
   If both are normal, pancreatitis unlikely
   If lipase elevated and normal amylase, consider hyperlipidemia
   If elevated amylase with normal lipase, consider macroamylasemia.

Plain Film of the Abdomen Shows:
  Absence of air under the diaphragm (perforation of ulcer or other viscus unlikely).
  Stomach dilated and displaced anteriorly, dilated loop of small intestine and colon cutoff sign, diagnosis of pancreatitis most likely.
  Calcifications of the midabdomen, compatible with recurrent chronic pancreatitis.

electrolytes, and plasma. It also might assist in the decision for early surgical or endoscopic intervention. Several prognostic scoring systems have been proposed that would allow such risk stratification. These systems are also useful in the comparison of outcomes between different series and in the evaluation of new modalities of treatment.

The outcome of acute pancreatitis appears to be most influenced by the severity of the attack. The cause is also important, since higher mortality is observed in idiopathic pancreatitis and when there is associated biliary tract disease. A higher mortality also is observed during the first attack of pancreatitis compared with subsequent attacks, regardless of cause.

To add objective laboratory criteria to the general guidelines, Ranson et al analyzed 43 early clinical and laboratory objective findings in 100 patients with acute pancreatitis, and identified 11 features that correlated with a complicated course or death.[8] Five of these signs could be determined on admission, and the remaining six during the subsequent 48 hours (Table 4.2). Notably, the level of serum amylase on admission is of no prognostic value.

When these factors were used subsequently in a prospective study of 200 patients, a severe course was correctly anticipated in 92.5% of the cases. Of 162 patients with less than 3 factors, only 1 proved to have severe disease.[9] Of the remaining 38

TABLE 4.2. **Early Clinical Prognostic Signs of Acute Pancreatitis**

At Admission or Diagnosis	During Initial 48 Hours
Age >55 years	Hematocrit fall >10% points
White blood cell count >16,000/μL	BUN level rise >5 mg/dL (1.79 mmol/L)
Blood glucose level >200 mg/dL (10 mmol/L)	Serum calcium level <8 mg/dL (2 mmol/L)
	Arterial PO_2 level <60 mm Hg (8 kPa)
Serum LDH >350 IU/L	Base deficit >4 mEq/L (4 mmol/L)
Serum (AST) GOT >250 IU/L	Estimated fluid sequestration >6000 mL

LDH, lactic dehydrogenase; GOT, glutamic oxaloacetic transaminase; AST, aspartate aminotransferase; BUN, blood urea nitrogen.
From Ranson JHC, Pasternack BS. Statistical methods for quantifying the severity of clinical pancreatitis. *J Surg Res* 1977;22:79–91.

patients with 3 or more risk factors, 24 had major complications or died. Subsequent studies by Jacobs et al[10] and Imrie et al[11] used comparable criteria with slight modifications and came to similar conclusions. Later Imrie's group reported that their scoring system correctly predicted severity in 79% of 405 episodes of pancreatitis.[12] It should be noted that in Ranson et al's series, patients were predominantly male alcoholics.[8] In Imrie et al's report, female patients with biliary disease were predominant.[11]

Another study using a more invasive approach that included peritoneal lavage was analyzed by Cooper et al.[13] They observed that hypotension (blood pressure <100 mm Hg), persistent hypocalcemia (<2 mmol/L), hypoxemia (PaO_2<60 mm Hg) and aspiration of more than 10 mL of "toxic broth" or dark fluid after lavage identified severe cases with an 84% diagnostic accuracy. In most centers around the world, there is considerable reservation about the use of diagnostic peritoneal lavage under these circumstances and this approach has not gained popularity in the United States. If ascites is present and brown and hemorrhagic fluid is aspirated, however, the prognosis is extremely grave.

Is there a single laboratory test that might assist in predicting the severity of pancreatitis? There has been a long search for a single test that will help in the early evaluation of acute pancreatitis and discrimination of the severe cases. For instance, the presence of methemalbumin has been demonstrated to be specific for hemorrhagic pancreatitis. The appearance of methemalbumin in the blood may take 72 or more hours, however, which obviously limits its value as an early indicator. A similar disadvantage has been observed with plasma concentration of fibrinogen, which has been observed to increase slowly during episodes of severe pancreatitis.

Measurement of C-reactive protein (CRP) appears to provide promising results. CRP is a glycoprotein that showed a distinct increase in one group of patients with acute necrotising pancreatitis compared with those with edematous pancreatitis.[14] The test is simple and can be performed quickly. It may prove to be as helpful as the multiple factor scoring systems in identifying severe forms of acute pancreatitis.

TABLE 4.3. Risk Factors in Acute Pancreatitis

Cardiac	Shock, tachycardia >130, arrhythmia, EKG changes
Pulmonary	Dyspnea, rales, PO_2 <60 mm Hg, adult respiratory distress syndrome
Renal	Urine output <50 mL/h, rising blood urea nitrogen and/or creatinine
Metabolic	Low or falling calcium, pH; albumin decrease
Hematologic	Falling hematocrit, diffuse intravascular coagulation (low platelets, fibrin split products)
Neurologic	Irritability, confusion, localizing signs
Hemorrhagic disease	Signs or peritoneal tap
Tense abdominal distension	Severe ileus, fluid + +
Interpretation	More than 1 risk factor = severe (potentially lethal disease)

From Bank S, Wise L, Gersten M. Risk factors in acute pancreatitis. Am J Gastroenterol 1983;78:637–640.

TABLE 4.4. A Simplified Criterion to Assess Severity of Pancreatitis

	During initial 48 hours
Cardiac	BP <90 mm Hg
	Tachycardia >130/min
Pulmonary	Dyspnea
	PO_2 <60 mm Hg
Renal	Urinary output <50 mL/h
Metabolic	Calcium <8 mg/dL
	Albumin <3.2 g/dL

From Agarwal N, Pitchumoni CS. Simplified prognostic criteria in acute pancreatitis. Pancreas 1986;1:69–73.

CLINICAL FACTORS

Efforts to predict outcome in acute pancreatitis have centered on clinical data that reflect multiorgan involvement and are easier to remember at the bedside: One such criterion proposed by Bank et al[15] is shown on Table 4.3. When 75 patients were analyzed according to these criteria, the outcome was excellent when no risk factors were present. Mortality rates reached 56% in those patients with one or more positive criteria. A modification that combines clinical and laboratory data has been proposed by Agarwal and Pitchumoni[16] (Table 4.4).

All of these criteria can be assessed within a few hours of admission of a patient with acute pancreatitis. The main predictors of severity common to all these criteria are sustained hypotension, hypocalcemia, hypoxemia, and progressive renal and respiratory failure.

In the management of severe pancreatitis, it is important to know whether pancreatic necrosis or infection are present. This information should be discussed jointly among the medical–surgical team that is caring for the patient because it often influences the decision for operation. Assessment of pancreatic necrosis may be obtained by computed tomography (CT) with vascular enhancement (contrast-enhanced CT). The areas that do not enhance are presumed to be ischemic. The diagnosis of infection of the ischemic tissue is greatly simplified by CT-guided percutaneous needle aspiration. This is a safe procedure and Gram's stain and culture of the aspirate usually leads to an earlier diagnosis of infection (usually within the first 2 weeks) than that strictly based on clinical and laboratory indices.[17]

ENDOSCOPY IN ACUTE PANCREATITIS

Traditionally acute pancreatitis was believed to be a contraindication to the performance of endoscopic retrograde cholangiography and pancreatography (ERCP). It was believed that the performance of such a study would aggravate acute pancreatitis, since it is well known that diagnostic ERCP can provoke an attack of acute pancreatitis. In one series this occurred in 8% of all ERCPs.[18] There have been a number of patients who have had an ERCP performed in the setting of acute pancreatitis related to gallstones impacted in the ampulla of Vater, however, and endoscopic sphincterotomy resulted in considerable improvement in their clinical condition.

A controlled trial of urgent endoscopic sphincterotomy versus conservative treatment for acute pancreatitis caused by gallstones has been reported recently by Neoptolemos et al.[19] They reported that an endoscopic sphincterotomy resulted in a better outcome than conservative, conventional treatment for patients with severe biliary pancreatitis. This is despite the fact that in the group of patients undergoing ERCP and endoscopic sphincterotomy for common bile duct stones, stones were not found to be impacted at the ampulla. The study is flawed, however, because it is difficult to compare the group of patients who had ERCP and sphincterotomy with the control group (in whom a diagnostic endoscopic examination was not performed within 72 hours of admission). Moreover, these findings are in marked contrast to the outcome of patients who have undergone early surgery for biliary pancreatitis since these patients have not fared better than those who have been treated conservatively. One wonders if the beneficial effects of sphincterotomy are related to a decreased pressure on the pancreatic duct orifice (although there are probably distinct, separate sphincters around the bile and pancreatic duct openings) and whether endoscopic insertion of a pancreatic drain would not be safer and as beneficial. Enthusiasts strongly advocate the performance of an urgent ERCP in patients who have severe biliary pancreatitis, however, and if common bile duct stones are documented, an endoscopic sphincterotomy should follow. Nevertheless, most patients, even those with severe acute biliary pancreatitis, do well without any interventional therapy and ERCP should be performed only in those patients who do not improve or who deteriorate during the first 72 hours. Moreover, it should be emphasized that ERCP should be performed only by those with the skills to perform an endoscopic sphincterotomy also.

Patients who have probable nonbiliary causes for acute pancreatitis are unlikely to benefit from an ERCP during the acute attack and, therefore, unless biliary pancreatitis is suspected, there is no merit to this invasive test. A possible exception to this guideline is for those patients who sustain blunt trauma to their abdomens, in whom an acute pancreatic duct injury is suspected.

A number of studies have evaluated the use of an elective ERCP in patients who have recovered from a presentation of "idiopathic" acute pancreatitis. In this small group of patients in whom obvious causes (such as the presence of gallstones on ultrasonography, metabolic abnormalities, or alcohol ingestion) have been excluded, ERCP may be helpful when performed after resolution of the acute pancreatitis. The American College of Physicians advises that ERCP usually is not indicated for the evaluation of a single episode of acute pancreatitis.[20] For those with recurrent attacks of "idiopathic" pancreatitis, a significant rate of unsuspected lesions will be encountered, including common bile duct stones, ampullary stenosis, pancreas divisum, and more rarely, pancreatic carcinoma.

Endoscopic treatment options for recurrent acute pancreatitis depend on the nature of the presumed cause for these attacks. Endoscopic sphincterotomy is standard practice for patients who have had a cholecystectomy and are found to have common bile duct stones. Much more controversial, however, is the relationship between pancreas divisum and acute pancreatitis.[21] Some of these patients have had amelioration of recurrent attacks of pancreatitis by the placement of a stent through the minor papilla or the performance of an endoscopic sphincterotomy of the minor papilla (see Case Presentation). Similar procedures have been performed in patients who have abnormal manometric studies of the sphincter of Oddi (hypertensive sphincter of their pancreatic duct orifice) and some of these patients have had fewer recurrent attacks. Nonetheless the safety and efficacy of these procedures should be considered unproven, however, especially because there is concern that the placement of pancreatic stents may induce pancreatic duct changes that mimic those of chronic pancreatitis. Such changes probably are reversible, however, in that they probably are related to stent blockage.

CASE PRESENTATION

> A 46-year-old woman was referred to our hospital with a history of five previous episodes of acute pancreatitis during the past 3 years. No gallstones or abnormalities of the common bile duct were found on two ultrasonographic studies and there was no history of alcoholism, drug ingestion, metabolic abnormalities, or family history of pancreatitis. Pancreatography was unsuccessful at an outside facility. At our institution a pancreatogram obtained through the major papilla revealed a narrowed short arborised duct that failed to extend to the body and tail of the pancreas. Pancreatography through a small accessory papilla showed a pancreatic duct of normal caliber and length that did not communicate with the major papilla. These findings are diagnostic of pancreas divisum (Fig. 4.2). No recurrence of acute pancreatitis occurred in a short follow-up period after endoscopic papillotomy of the minor papilla.

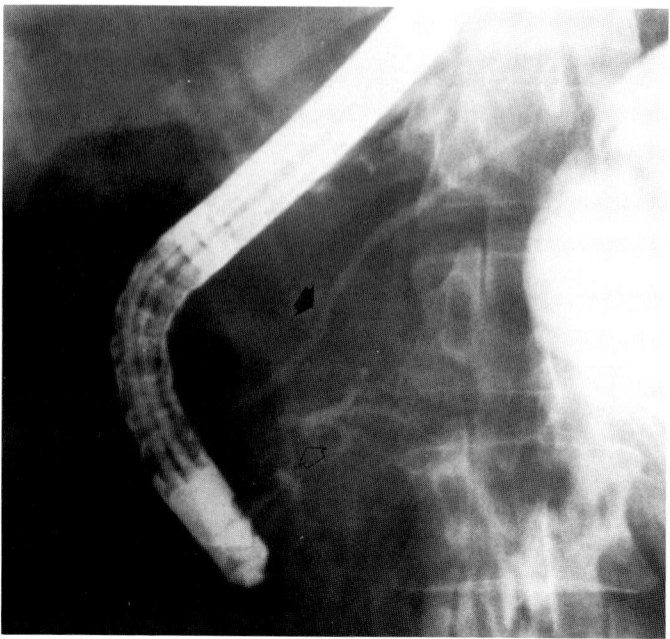

FIGURE 4.2. Pancreas divisum: Injection of contrast via major papilla demonstrates a rudimentary ventral pancreatic duct (open arrow). Contrast from previous injection through minor papilla shows main (dorsal) pancreatic duct (closed arrow). Note lack of communication between ventral and dorsal ducts.

In the absence of any other identifiable factor, pancreas divisum was believed to be the cause of the recurrent attacks of acute pancreatitis. The clinical course after papillotomy suggests, but does not confirm, this relationship. The follow-up period, however, has been too short.

References

1. Davidson BR, Neoptolemos JP, Leese T, et al. Biochemical prediction of gallstones in acute pancreatitis: a prospective study of three systems. *Br J Surg* 1988;75:213–215.
2. Van Gossum A, Seferian V, Rodzynck JJ, et al. Early detection of biliary pancreatitis. *Dig Dis Sci* 1984;29:97–101.
3. Spechler SJ, Dalton JW, Robbins AH, et al. Prevalence of normal serum amylase levels in patients with acute alcoholic pancreatitis. *Dig Dis Sci* 1983;28:865–869.
4. Steinberg WM, Goldstein SS, Davis ND, et al. Diagnostic assays in acute pancreatitis. *Ann Intern Med* 1985;102:576–580.
5. Cherry IS, Crandall LA, Jr. The specificity of pancreatic lipase: its appearance in the blood after pancreatic injury. *Am J Physiol* 1932;100:266–273.
6. Roberts IM, Mercer D. Radioimmunoassay for human pancreatic lipase in acute pancreatitis. *Dig Dis Sci* 1987;32:388–392.
7. Kolars JC, Ellis CJ, Levitt MD. Comparison of serum amylase pancreatic isoamylase and lipase in patients with hyperamylasemia. *Dig Dis Sci* 1984;29:289–293.

8. Ranson JHC, Rifkind KM, Roses DF, et al. Prognostic signs and the role of operative management in acute pancreatitis. *Surg Gynecol Obstet* 1974;139:69–81.
9. Ranson JHC, Pasternack BS. Statistical methods for quantifying the severity of clinical acute pancreatitis. *J Surg Res* 1977;22:79–91.
10. Jacobs ML, Daggett WM, Civetta JM, et al. Acute pancreatitis: analysis of factors influencing survival. *Ann Surg* 1977;185:43–51.
11. Imrie CW, Benjamin IS, Ferguson JC, et al. A single centre double blind trial of trasylol therapy in primary acute pancreatitis. *Br J Surg* 1978;65:337–341.
12. Blamey SL, Imrie CW, O'Neill J, et al. Prognostic factors in acute pancreatitis. *Gut* 1984; 25:1340–1346.
13. Cooper MJ, Williamson RCN, Pollock AV. The role of peritoneal lavage in the prediction and treatment of severe acute pancreatitis. *Ann R Coll Surg Engl* 1982;64:422–427.
14. Wilson C, Heads A, Shenkin A, Imrie CW. C-reactive protein, antiproteases and complement factors as objective markers of severity in acute pancreatitis. *Br J Surg* 1989; 76:177–181.
15. Bank S, Wise L, Gersten M. Risk factors in acute pancreatitis. *Am J Gastroenterol* 1983; 78:637–640.
16. Agarwal N, Pitchumoni CS. Simplified prognostic criteria in acute pancreatitis. *Pancreas* 1986;1:69–73.
17. Banks PA, Gerzof SG, Chong FK, et al. Bacteriologic status of necrotic tissue in necrotizing pancreatitis. *Pancreas* 1990;5:330–333.
18. LaFerla G, Gordon S, Archibald M, et al. Hyperamylasaemia and acute pancreatitis following endoscopic retrogade cholangiopancreatography. *Pancreas* 1986;1:160–163.
19. Neoptolemos JP, London NJ, James D, et al. Controlled trial of urgent endoscopic retrograde cholangiopancreatography and endoscopic sphincterotomy versus conservative treatment for acute pancreatitis due to gallstones. *Lancet* 1988;2:979–983.
20. Health and Public Policy Committee, American College of Physicians. Clinical competence in diagnostic endoscopic retrograde cholangiopancreatography. *Ann Int Med* 1988; 108:142–144.
21. Cotton PB. Pancreas divisum. *Pancreas* 1988;3:245–247.

Chapter 5

Imaging Studies in Acute Pancreatitis

PHILIP W. RALLS

RADIOLOGY IN ACUTE PANCREATITIS

Conventional radiographic techniques have limited use in the diagnosis and management of acute pancreatitis. Generally speaking, these procedures merely detect nonspecific findings associated with the disease. Chest radiographs may be useful in patients with pulmonary symptoms. The most frequent findings are pleural effusions and atelectasis. Plain abdominal films, consisting of an antero-posterior, plus either an upright or left-lateral decubitus film, may prove useful and are probably warranted in all patients with suspected pancreatitis. Calcifications from chronic pancreatitis may be detected. Ascites, stomach, small bowel, and colonic dilation (Fig. 5.1), and occasionally a mass indicative of abscess or pseudocyst may be identified. The former findings are nonspecific. Detection of free intraperitoneal air may be helpful in diagnosing perforated peptic ulcer. Contrast studies (upper gastrointestinal series, barium enema) are rarely indicated, having been largely supplanted by imaging techniques—real-time sonography and computed tomography (CT). Magnetic resonance imaging is virtually useless in acute pancreatitis because it is difficult to perform in uncooperative, critically ill patients, lacks a satisfactory gastrointestinal contrast agent, is cumbersome at best in guiding percutaneous diagnostic and therapeutic procedures, and is much more expensive than CT or sonography.[1,2]

Because acute pancreatitis is generally diagnosed on clinical and laboratory grounds, imaging is rarely required early in the disease. The only exception is sonography. Real-time sonography is often useful in detecting gallstones, a frequent cause of acute pancreatitis. Of special importance is the detection of bile duct dilation related to common duct stones, since early intervention may be necessary when calculous common duct obstruction is present.

In many patients with mild acute pancreatitis, CT and sonography are completely normal. Sonographic findings, when present, may include pancreatic edema and peripancreatic inflammatory changes. The sonograms reveal hypoechoic enlargement of the pancreas or decreased echogenicity in the peripancreatic–retroperitoneal re-

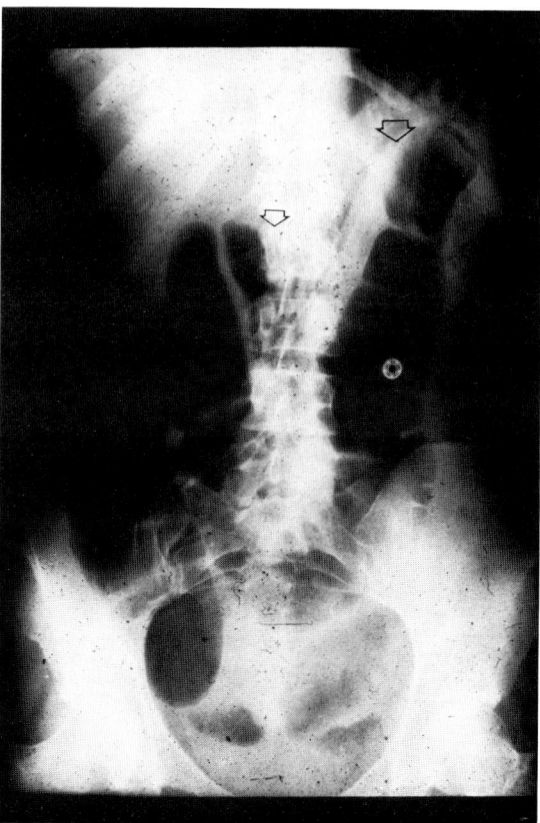

FIGURE 5.1. Plain film of the abdomen showing distension of the ascending and right side of the transverse colon with an abrupt "cutoff" of the gas (between arrows) at the left side of the transverse colon.

gions (Fig. 5.2). Increased echogenicity may occur when hemorrhagic pancreatitis is present.[3]

Because acute pancreatitis often causes dilated air-filled bowel loops, sonographic imaging of the pancreas may be difficult. Careful technique including scanning through the flanks and oral water administration to fill overlying gastrointestinal tract structures may allow adequate visualization.

When it is abnormal, CT in acute pancreatitis reveals a diffusely enlarged pancreas of decreased density. Focal alterations in parenchymal shape and density are less common. Occasionally, a dilated pancreatic duct (3 mm or greater in internal diameter) may be detected. Peripancreatic abnormalities, usually increased density of the peripancreatic fat, may occur (Fig. 5.3). If the illness worsens, contrast-enhanced CT scan will identify perfused areas of the pancreas whereas poorly perfused areas, which may represent necrotic tissue or fluid material, will enhance to a lesser degree. Peripancreatic exudates (phlegmon), fluid collections, or hemorrhage may be detected.

In addition, percutaneous guided aspiration is successful in distinguishing severe sterile pancreatitis from pancreatic infection and may help to avoid unnecessary sur-

IMAGING STUDIES

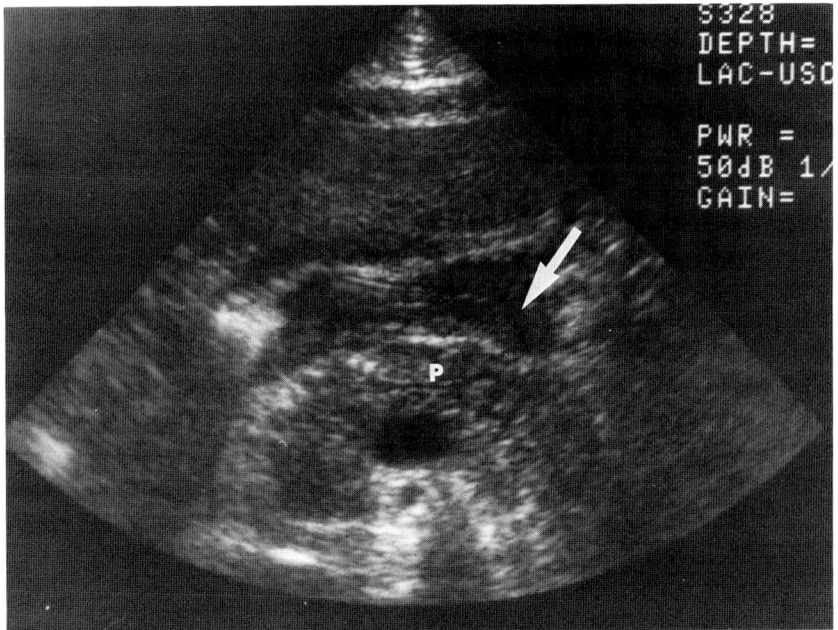

FIGURE 5.2. Transverse sonogram of the body of the pancreas (P). A hypoechoic region of phlegmon (arrow) is noted ventral to the pancreas, which is of normal echogenicity.

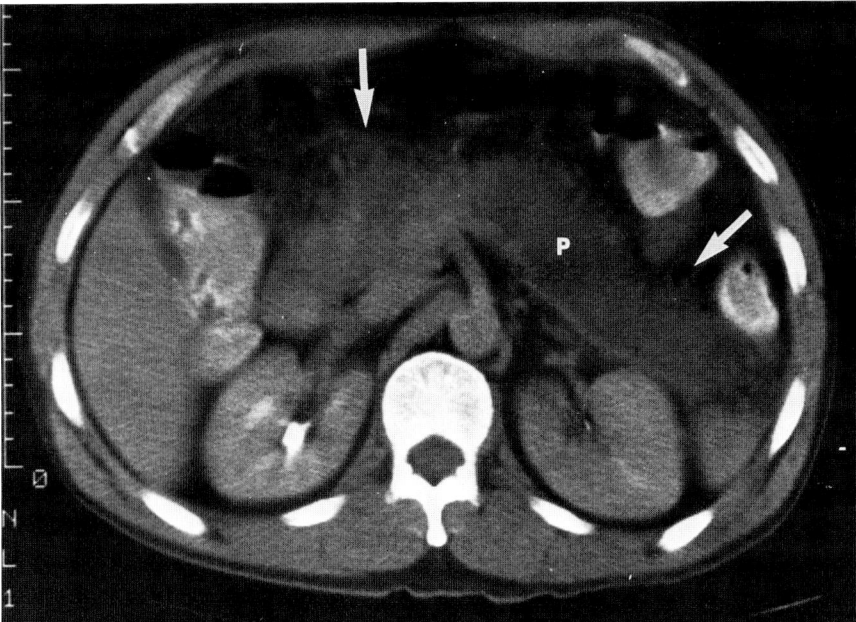

FIGURE 5.3. Transverse CT of the body and tail of the pancreas (P). Note the decreased density of the pancreas and the extrapancreatic inflammatory change (arrows).

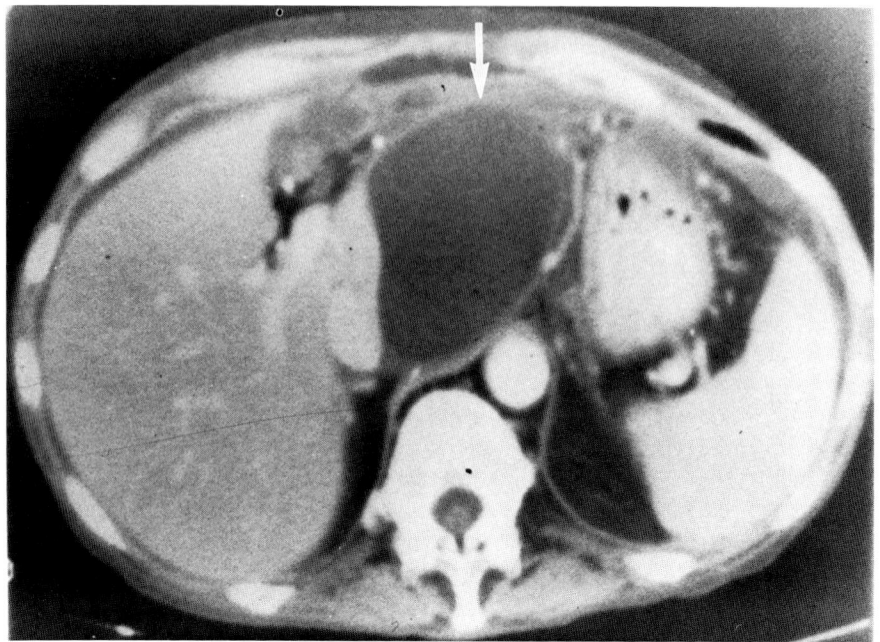

FIGURE 5.4. Transverse CT showing a large pancreatic pseudocyst (arrow).

gery. Furthermore, percutaneous intervention provides an alternative therapeutic modality. After a diagnostic needle aspiration with a 20-gauge or 22-gauge needle, a catheter can be inserted to drain pseudocysts or infected pseudocysts. If patients are properly selected by an experienced gastroenterologist–surgeon–radiologist team, percutaneous guided drainage may eliminate the need for surgery in as many as 80% of patients. The following case presentation is illustrative.

Case Presentation

A 26-year-old man with a previous episode of alcohol-related pancreatitis was discharged asymptomatic 3 weeks ago. He was readmitted with new onset of nausea and vomiting and complaining of severe constant midepigastric pain radiated to the back. The patient denied any recent fever, chills, hematemesis, or melena although he claimed to have lost 3 kg in the last 3 weeks. On admission vomiting was frequent, initially greenish and later pinkish, and strongly positive for occult blood. Physical examination except for tachycardia, moderate epigastric tenderness, and sucussion splash, was negative. A nasogastric tube was placed and 2L of aspirate recovered. Aspiration was continued and an ultrasound of the pancreas done (Fig. 5.4). A large pancreatic fluid collection was visualized. Needle aspiration revealed fluid with a high amylase content (12,000 U/dL) without white cells or bacteria and the culture was negative. A pig-tail catheter was inserted under ultrasound (US) guidance (Fig. 5.5).

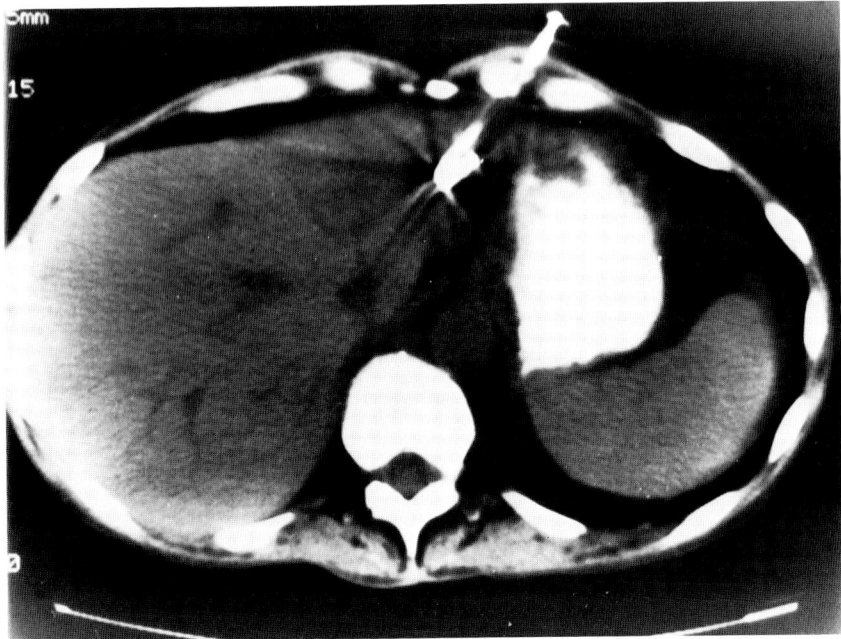

FIGURE 5.5. Transverse CT showing marked reduction of the pancreatic pseudocyst.

The collection decreased in size, the symptoms and signs subsided, feeding was restarted 3 weeks after admission, and the patient was discharged after 4 weeks of treatment.[4]

Percutaneous guided drainage may also constitute an alternative nonsurgical modality for many infected pseudocysts.

The main use of CT and sonography in acute pancreatitis is to seek potential complications. These include hemorrhage, retroperitoneal exudate (phlegmon), pseudocyst, and abscess. Obtaining sonographic images of the peripancreatic region may be difficult since dilated gas-filled bowel loops may obscure the pancreas. Although sonography is far from useless, CT is preferred when seeking complications of pancreatitis because it is not limited by bone or gas. Although real-time sonography can detect both phlegmon and fluid collections, CT is usually superior in both detection of fluid collections and in determining extent of disease. CT is most useful in critically ill patients. Sonography is best for studying known pseudocysts in relatively healthy patients since it is noninvasive and inexpensive.[5]

A critical factor in selecting an imaging modality to assess pancreatitis patients is the ability to guide percutaneous diagnostic aspiration and therapeutic drainage. Image and clinical findings alone rarely permit confident differentiation between bland fluid collections and pancreatic abscess. Percutaneous image-guided aspiration can achieve this without surgery. Either CT or sonography can be used to guide diagnostic aspiration or percutaneous pseudocyst drainage. When placing a drainage catheter in a fluid collection, CT is preferred if there is a question of intervening bowel.

References

1. Balthazar EJ. CT diagnosis and staging of acute pancreatitis. *Radiol Clin North Am* 1989; 27:19–37.
2. Vernacchia FS, Jeffrey RB, Federle MP, et al. Pancreatic abscess: predictive value of early abdominal CT. *Radiology* 1987;162:435–438.
3. Jeffrey RB, Laing FC, Wing VW. Extrapancreatic spread of acute pancreatitis: new observations with real-time ultrasound. *Radiology* 1986;159:707–711.
4. Van Sonnenberg E, Casola G, Varney RR, et al. Imaging and interventional radiology for pancreatitis and its complications. *Radiol Clin North Am* 1989; 27:65–72.
5. Nuutinen P, Kivisaari L, Sehroder T. Contrast-enhanced computed tomography and microangiography of the pancreas in acute human hemorrhagic/necrotizing pancreatitis. *Pancreas* 1988;3:53–60.

Chapter 6

Management of Acute Pancreatitis

JORGE E. VALENZUELA

In spite of the progress in our understanding of pancreatic cell biology and physiology and information gained from experimental models of pancreatitis, the medical management of acute pancreatitis remains basically supportive. The principal goals in treating a patient with acute pancreatitis are to provide pain relief and to correct fluid and electrolyte disturbances.

ANALGESIA

Once the diagnosis has been established, strong analgesia should be provided. This requires the use of opiates such as morphine 8 to 15 mg or meperidine (Demerol HCL) 50 to 100 mg every 4 to 6 hours intramuscularly (IM) or intravenously (IV) in doses sufficient to alleviate the pain. Hydroxyzine HCL (Vistaril) 25 to 100 mg IM may be added in agitated alcoholic patients with persistent nausea and vomiting. The theoretical consideration that some of these drugs increase the sphincter of Oddi pressure should not preclude their use. There is no clinical evidence to suggest that they aggravate the severity of an attack.

CORRECTION OF FLUID AND ELECTROLYTE DISTURBANCES

Depletion of intravascular volume is the result of vomiting, third space losses, peripancreatic and peritoneal exudate, and bleeding (in cases of hemorrhagic pancreatitis). Vigorous intravenous fluid administration should be started as soon as possible to restore intravascular volume, and correct acid–base and electrolyte imbalances. Large volumes (3 to 5 L or more in the first 24 hours) may be required. Careful monitoring of vital signs, hourly urinary output, sequential determinations of serum electrolytes, blood urea nitrogen (BUN), serum creatinine and in most cases, arterial blood gases should be done. Hypovolemia, ischemia, and shock are among the factors that often cause diffuse multisystem parenchymal damage and determine early mortality and complications. Thus the restoration of intravascular volume is the most important early therapeutic effort with a significant impact on prognosis.

In some instances plasma and blood transfusions are necessary to maintain serum albumin levels over 2.5 gm/dL and hematocrit over 30%. There is no conclusive evidence that colloid solutions improve outcome when they are given routinely, however. A baseline electrocardiogram and chest roentgenogram are recommended particularly in elderly patients. As fluids are administered vigorously, monitoring central venous pressure may be indicated whenever overload is feared.

In patients with severe pancreatitis, hypocalcemia may require parenteral calcium administration. The amount should be determined by serial calcium measurements. Hypomagnesemia, especially in chronic alcoholics, may also require treatment. Recognition and treatment of low serum calcium levels is important for two reasons. Serious cardiac arrhythmias could occur. The prognosis and severity of the pancreatitis is related to the degree of hypocalcemia. Thus, patients with serum calcium levels less than 7.8 mg/dL have lesser chances to survive.

A brief period of systolic and diastolic hypertension has been documented in acute pancreatitis.[1] The cause is unclear, but it may be related to the release of an unknown factor from the pancreas. Often this finding is missed because patients consult their physician late or the loss of volume compensates. It is important to be aware of this syndrome because patients may be normotensive in spite of severe hypovolemia; then a lack of volume replacement could have adverse consequences on renal function.

Hypoxemia that requires oxygen administration occurs in 25% to 30% of patients. Because the onset may be insidious and can be present even in those with disease of only moderate severity, arterial blood gases should be monitored in most patients every 12 hours for the first few days. Supplemental O_2 therapy should be given when the PaO_2 is less than 70 mm Hg. Occasionally, especially in patients with severe pancreatitis, a form of adult respiratory distress syndrome develops. Then endotracheal intubation and mechanical ventilation may be required.

Antibiotics are of no proven value in the typical case of acute pancreatitis. They should be used for the treatment of specific suppurative complications, and chosen on the basis of culture and sensitivity data when possible. Nevertheless, in patients with hemorrhagic, necrotizing pancreatitis, it is common to try broad-spectrum antibiotics to decrease the chance for the development of pancreatic abscess. The efficacy of this approach is unproved.

ENDOSCOPY IN ACUTE PANCREATITIS

The role of endoscopic treatment of acute biliary pancreatitis has been reviewed in Chapter 4.

SUPPRESSION OF PANCREATIC SECRETION

Based on the assumption that acute pancreatitis results from enzymatic "autodigestion," the aims of therapy have been directed to suppress the synthesis and secretion of enzymes. Other techniques have also been considered. Oral intake is prohibited, and a nasogastric tube is inserted except in the mildest of cases; this situation is observed most commonly in chronic alcoholics with recurrent episodes of pancreatitis. The goal is to aspirate gastric secretions, and to avoid the release of secretin and cholecystokinin (CCK) that would occur if these fluids entered the duodenum. The most important benefit probably derives from the elimination of vomiting and abdominal distention that would otherwise occur in these patients when intestinal ileus is generally present. Feeding is usually resumed when peristalsis has returned, pain is gone, and the serum enzyme abnormalities are normal. Resumption of diet has to be determined carefully because in some instances it causes a flare-up of the disease, and one must wait longer.

Inhibition of Pancreatic Enzyme Synthesis

Since 5-fluorouracil (5-FU) inhibits DNA, RNA, and pancreatic enzyme synthesis, a role for 5-FU in the therapy of acute pancreatitis has been proposed. Experimental and uncontrolled clinical trials suggest that 5-FU has beneficial effects in the course of acute pancreatitis. When this effect was tested in one controlled study, however, 5-FU was no more effective than placebo in significantly reducing mortality rate, length of hospital stay, and incidence of complications. Patients that received 5-FU had less pain, however, the dose of 5-FU given in this study, 250 mg per 24 hours in a single dose, was lower than that used in treatment of malignancies and caused no apparent side effects.[2] No further clinical controlled trials have been conducted with 5-FU since some reservation exists in the medical community about the drug's potential toxicity.

Inhibition of Acinar Cell Secretion

Inhibition of acinar cell secretion can be achieved by suppressing stimuli elicited by food intake and by blocking the hormonal and neural mechanisms that transmit the stimulation to the exocrine pancreas.

Cimetidine

When gastric acid reaches the intestine, secretin is released, which stimulates pancreatic secretion. Since cimetidine inhibits acid secretion, it was proposed that it could have beneficial effects in the treatment of pancreatitis. Controlled prospective trials have shown no significant differences between patients receiving cimetidine and controls in terms of clinical course and complications, however.[3] In fact some patients receiving cimetidine had a longer elevation in the serum amylase level. Studies in rats have actually suggested that pancreatitis could be caused by cimetidine administration, although no clinical cases of cimetidine-induced pancreatitis have been reported. Thus, there appears to be no role for cimetidine therapy in the management of acute pancreatitis.

CCK Blockers

CCK plays an important role in the stimulation of enzyme secretion. A role for excessive release of CCK in the pathogenesis of pancreatitis has not been proven, although supramaximal doses of cerulein, a CCK-analogue, induces pancreatitis in rats. A number of CCK antagonists exist (eg, proglumide, asperlicin, L-364,718) that are potent inhibitors of the physiologic effects of CCK. In animal models of pancreatitis, amelioration has been observed after administration of these drugs (usually before the pancreatitis has become established). Clinical trials with these new compounds are not yet available.

Inhibitors of Pancreatic Secretion

Peptides such as glucagon and somatostatin that inhibit pancreatic enzyme secretion in experimental animals and in humans have been proposed in the therapy of acute pancreatitis. Randomized controlled studies have failed to demonstrate the efficacy of either peptide in patients with pancreatitis, however.[4]

Anticholinergics

Acetylcholine appears to be the main neurotransmitter of gastropancreatic and enteropancreatic reflexes, since at least 50% of the postprandial pancreatic secretory response is suppressed in animals and humans after administration of atropine. More than 4 decades ago the use of atropine in the management of acute pancreatitis was proposed, and it was adopted widely initially. When the efficacy of this anticholinergic was properly evaluated in prospective studies, however, no significant differences in the clinical course of patients receiving the drug was observed.[5] In addition, the use of anticholinergics has some adverse effects. They cause tachycardia, aggravation of ileus, urinary retention, and constipation. Thus, the routine use of anticholinergics in the management of acute pancreatitis has been abandoned.

Inactivation of Enzymes

The proteases, lipases, and vasoactive compounds released in the vicinity of the pancreas and into the general circulation are believed to play a major role in the local and systemic manifestations of pancreatitis. Removal or inactivation of these enzymes has been attempted.

Peritoneal Lavage

It was reasoned that removal of active pancreatic enzymes from the ascitic fluid could favorably modify the course of acute pancreatitis. Initial clinical trials of peritoneal lavage showed encouraging results and its use was recommended in patients with severe pancreatitis. One multicenter, randomized, controlled trial tested the efficacy of therapeutic peritoneal lavage in more than 90 patients with severe acute pancreatitis. They concluded that peritoneal lavage did not modify the survival rate, the incidence of pancreatic collections, or serum enzyme levels.[6] The lack of beneficial effect of peritoneal lavage in severe pancreatitis was subsequently confirmed by another prospective study that included 39 patients with severe acute pancreatitis. Peritoneal dialysis did not affect any of the prognostic signs, nor the clinical course of the disease. As expected, the amylase concentration in the peritoneal fluid was significantly reduced.[7] From these two studies it might be concluded that peritoneal lavage does not seem to add any benefit to the treatment of acute pancreatitis, although there is some suggestion that long-term lavage (7 days) may be beneficial in reducing the incidence of pancreatic sepsis and mortality rates in a small group of patients.[8]

Enzyme Inhibitors

Inhibition of tryptic activity was postulated as an effective method to reduce the inflammation in acute pancreatitis. Aprotinin (Trasylol), a protease inhibitor, was introduced in the 1950s and there were initial enthusiastic reports about its use in experimental pancreatitis as well as in some early clinical trials. Several subsequent prospective controlled trials failed to demonstrate any benefit in regard to the course of acute pancreatitis, complication rate, and survival.[9] The use of aprotinin has been completely abandoned.

Two synthetic proteinase inhibitors, gabexate mesilate (FOY) and camostate (FOY-305), have become available. These compounds have a broader spectrum of actions since they effectively inhibit trypsin, plasmin, kallikrein, thrombin, and to a certain degree phospholipase A activity. A favorable effect on severe experimental pancreatitis has been reported, but there are, as of yet, no clinical experiences with either.

Phospholipase A_2 is present in high concentrations in the human pancreas. Elevated levels of this enzyme are detected in the serum of patients with acute pancreatitis and a pathogenetic role has been proposed for it. Thus, phospholipase A_2 inhibitors (eg, cytidine diphosphate choline and Ca Na_2 EDTA) have been tested in a few patients with acute pancreatitis, with apparent improvement in the clinical course.[10] Controlled prospective studies with larger number of patients are needed. Observations of possible beneficial effects with administration of anesthetics (eg, xylocaine) in experimental pancreatitis are related to inhibition of phospholipases. No clinical evaluation of the anesthetics in the treatment of patients with pancreatitis is available.

The overall analysis of all the different modalities in the medical treatment of acute pancreatitis reveals that none appear to offer any additional benefit in the management of this disease. These failures may be due to several factors. First, the outcome of pancreatitis and the variable degrees of severity may be affected by the different causes. Second, clinical trials have not included a number of patients large enough to analyze a population with comparable severity. Large multicenter trials should be designed to gather comparable numbers of patients and to provide sufficient statistical power. Third, duration of the treatment should be extended at least to 2 weeks, because severe acute pancreatitis seems to have two peaks of morbidity and mortality. The first peak occurs early and seems to be related to systemic manifestations. A second peak occurs after the second week and appears to be related to the formation of pancreatic and peripancreatic collections and infections.[11]

References

1. Sankaran S, Lucas CE, Walt AJ. Transient hypertension with acute pancreatitis. *Surg Gynecol Obstet* 1974;138:235–238.
2. Saario IA. 5-Fluorouracil the treatment of acute pancreatitis. *Am J Surg* 1983; 145:349–352.
3. Broe PJ, Zinner MJ, Cameron JL. A clinical trial of cimetidine in acute pancreatitis. *Surg Gynecol Obstet* 1982;154:13–16.
4. Usadel KH, Uberla KK, Leuschner U. Treatment of acute pancreatitis with somatostatin: results of a multicenter double-blind trial. *Dig Dis Sci* 1985;30:992. Abstract.
5. Cameron JL, Mehigan D, Zuidema GD. Evaluation of atropine in acute pancreatitis. *Surg Gynecol Obstet* 1979;148:206–208.
6. Mayer AD, McMahon MJ, Corfield AP, et al. Controlled clinical trial of peritoneal lavage for the treatment of severe acute pancreatitis. *N Engl J Med* 1985;312:399–404.
7. Ihse, I, Evander A, Holmberg JT, et al. Influence of peritoneal lavage on objective prognostic signs in acute pancreatitis. *Ann Surg* 1986;204:122–127.
8. Ranson JHC, Berman RS. Long peritoneal lavage decreases pancreatic sepsis in acute pancreatitis. *Ann Surg* 1990;211:708–716.
9. Imrie CW, Benjamin IS, Ferguson JC, et al. A single-centre double-blind trial of trasylol therapy in primary acute pancreatitis. *Br J Surg* 1978;65:337–341.
10. Tykka, H, Mahlberg K, Pantzar P, et al. Phospholipase A_2 inhibitors and their possible clincial use in the treatment of acute pancreatitis. *Scand J Gastroent* 1980;15:519–528.
11. Steinberg WM, Schlesselman SE. Treatment of acute pancreatitis. *Gastroenterology* 1987; 93:1420–1427.

Chapter 7

Local Complications of Pancreatitis Including Pseudocyst and Ascites

HOWARD A. REBER
H. GILL CRYER

PANCREATIC ABSCESS

Pancreatic abscess complicates about 5% of all cases of acute pancreatitis. It is more likely to occur in hemorrhagic or necrotizing pancreatitis, and is an especially frequent complication of postoperative pancreatitis. Although the term "abscess" generally refers to an encapsulated collection of purulent material regardless of its site, it has a broader meaning in the present context. Thus, although purulent collections do develop, often the diagnosis is made and treatment instituted when the pancreas and peripancreatic tissue are infected but there is no pus. This has been called an infected pancreatic phlegmon. The terms abscess and infected phlegmon have been used interchangeably.[1]

The source of the invading organisms is uncertain. They probably come from the adjacent colon and are believed to pass through the colonic wall, which has been made abnormally permeable by the nearby inflammation. Another possible source is the biliary tree. There is no evidence that prophylactic antibiotics given early in the course of pancreatitis decrease the incidence of pancreatic abscess.

Clinical Findings

Pancreatic infection should be suspected when a patient with acute pancreatitis fails to improve after a week of the usual therapy, or when clinical deterioration develops the second or third week after initial improvement. There is recent evidence that the infection actually occurs by the end of the first week of the disease in many patients, but the diagnosis and treatment have typically been delayed an additional 1 to 3 weeks. Usually there is a rising fever (39 to 40°C) and leucocytosis (15,000 to 20,000/μL). But many patients may have only a low-grade temperature (37.5 to

38.5°C) and a white blood cell count less than 10,000/μL. Nausea, vomiting, vague epigastric pain, tenderness, and a palpable mass may be present. The serum amylase is usually normal, but the alkaline phosphatase is elevated and the serum albumin is often below 2.5 g/dL. There may be a pleural effusion, which is characteristically sterile, with normal amylase concentration. Plain radiographs of the abdomen or computed tomography (CT) scans rarely show gas bubbles in the region of the pancreas, which are diagnostic of infection (the gas is a product of bacterial metabolism and fermentation). More commonly, however, CT scans reveal an edematous pancreas with fluid collections in the peripancreatic area. These should be sampled using percutaneous needle aspiration, guided by CT or ultrasound techniques.[2] If Gram's stain or culture of the material reveals organisms, the diagnosis is established.

Recent studies stress the value of contrast-enhanced CT examinations in this setting.[3] A standard CT scan is obtained, followed by the rapid injection of intravenous contrast material. Then the scan is repeated. Normally perfused structures appear more dense in this second scan. When portions of the pancreas do not enhance in this way, they are considered to be necrotic. Because the necrotic areas are more likely to be infected, this information has been used to help choose the site for needle aspiration. One group has even recommended surgical intervention without proof of infection when more than half of the pancreas appears nonviable by this technique.[1] The value of such an approach is uncertain.

Treatment

As soon as the diagnosis of pancreatic infection is certain, surgical exploration is mandatory. In some cases when the patient is deteriorating clinically in spite of apparently adequate medical treatment, surgery may be indicated even if it has not been possible to prove infection. Percutaneous drainage of the infection is almost never an acceptable alternative because of the multiloculated nature of these abscesses and the fact that they typically contain thick particulate material. This would rapidly plug these small drainage catheters. Patients should receive broad-spectrum antibiotics preoperatively, chosen to provide activity against a variety of enteric organisms (*Escherichia coli, Bacteroides, Klebsiella, Proteus*). Antibiotics must be considered as an adjunct to surgical drainage, however; they are inadequate therapy by themselves.

Infected and necrotic material should be debrided through a wide abdominal incision. External drainage is accomplished through large sump drains laid down to the pancreatic bed and other involved areas. Because the infection typically spreads through the retroperitoneal tissue planes, these areas may extend some distance from the pancreas (eg, behind the right or left colon, into the pelvis). Postoperative peritoneal lavage through catheters placed at this time may also have some value.[4,5]

These patients often require additional operations to drain recurrent abscesses that may develop before the infection is eradicated completely. A hospitalization of several months duration is common. Even at discharge many patients still have external drainage tubes in place that continue to drain particulate debris, pancreatic juice, or both for many months.

The prognosis for patients with pancreatic abscess is grave. The mortality rate is 30%, a consequence of several factors.[6,7] The diagnosis is difficult to make and is often made late in the course of the illness (see Chapter 4). Surgical drainage is often incomplete, and the need for reoperation may not be appreciated.

PANCREATIC PSEUDOCYST

Pancreatic pseudocysts are encapsulated collections of fluid with high concentrations of pancreatic enzymes that arise from the pancreas. They complicate about 2% of cases of acute pancreatitis and occur singly in about 85% of cases. Pseudocysts are usually located within or adjacent to the pancreas in the lesser peritoneal sac, but they also are found distant from this site (eg, neck, mediastinum, pelvis). This happens when the fluid dissects through retroperitoneal tissue planes before a cyst develops. The wall of the pseudocyst is not lined by true epithelium. It consists of an inflammatory fibrous membrane formed from the peritoneal, mesenteric, and serosal surfaces that limit its spread as the lesion develops.

Pseudocysts develop in two different clinical settings and their pathogenesis is somewhat different in each.[8] In the first setting the cyst is a complication of an episode of acute pancreatitis that becomes evident as the inflammatory process evolves. There is an accumulation of edema fluid and extravasation of pancreatic juice, perhaps in association with pancreatic ductal rupture. The fluid is not reabsorbed as the inflammation resolves, and a cyst develops. In the second setting the cyst develops silently in a patient with chronic pancreatitis, and there is no preceding episode of acute inflammation. The mechanism is believed to be secondary to ductal obstruction with dilation of the obstructed ductal segment. Eventually a retention cyst is formed that loses its epithelial lining as it enlarges. It is important clinically to make the distinction between these two modes of development, since in the first case it is advisable to wait 4 to 6 weeks before definitive surgical treatment is undertaken. When the pseudocyst develops without an episode of acute inflammation, waiting is not necessary (see subsequent section on treatment).

Clinical Findings

A pseudocyst should be suspected in a patient with acute pancreatitis when the illness persists more than a week during optimal medical treatment, or when the clinical condition worsens after a period of recovery. Anorexia, nausea, vomiting, fever, weight loss, tenderness, and a palpable mass are present in half of the cases. Over 85% of patients with pseudocysts complain of abdominal pain. In patients in whom the cyst develops during an episode of acute pancreatitis, the pain may develop along with the pancreatitis or there may be a pain-free interval before the cyst is discovered. In patients with chronic pancreatitis in whom chronic pain has been a long-standing symptom, a pseudocyst is often heralded by the appearance of a different type of pain. Vomiting may be a sign of gastric or duodenal obstruction caused by compression of these structures by the cyst. A pseudocyst can also produce jaundice by compression of the common bile duct. Elevated serum amylase and moderate leukocytosis are present in half of the patients. When patients with acute pancreatitis have a persistent elevation in their serum amylase concentration for as long as 3 weeks, half have a pseudocyst.

Although most patients with a pseudocyst have a mass that distorts the stomach, duodenum or both on an upper gastrointestinal series, it is not possible to distinguish a cyst from an abscess or pancreatic phlegmon with this study. Ultrasound or CT scans can distinguish between a fluid-filled and a solid mass, and are useful in the diagnosis and management of pseudocysts. If a solid mass or phlegmon is found, it should be studied at intervals to determine whether cysts will develop within it, or until it resolves. If a cystic mass is found, repeated examinations are also indicated to plan treatment. Twenty to forty percent of acute pseudocysts resolve spontaneously as the inflammatory process resolves.[9] Then no further treatment is indicated. Most of the remainder require surgical management to treat the symptoms and avoid the development of complications.

Although endoscopic retrograde cholangiopancreatography (ERCP) examination may reveal the cyst and its communication with the pancreatic ductal system in 50% of cases, in most it is not necessary. ERCP should be done when the patient is jaundiced or there is an elevated alkaline phosphatase concentration in the serum to provide information about the common bile duct in relation to the cyst. It may be indicated in other circumstances when there are questions about the anatomy of the pancreatic and bile ducts in relation to the cyst. Multiple cysts are evident in 10% to 15% of cases. Because of the danger of introducing infection into the cyst with the ERCP, prophylactic antibiotics should be given before it, and it should only be performed within 24 hours of the time that elective surgery has been planned.

The relative value of ultrasound and CT scans for the diagnosis and management of pseudocysts has been debated. Because CT is more sensitive and specific, it should be used for the initial diagnosis so that an accurate image of the size, location, and number of cysts is known. Because of the radiation and higher cost associated with CT, the interval examinations should be done with ultrasound. Because of the availability of both of these techniques, small pseudocysts that would have previously escaped detection are being diagnosed. Asymptomatic cysts smaller than 5 cm probably do not require treatment.

Differential Diagnosis

In the clinical setting of acute pancreatitis, pseudocysts must be distinguished from pancreatic abscess. Patients with an abscess are usually more toxic, with a higher fever and leukocytosis. Occasionally it may be necessary to obtain fluid for Gram's stain and culture from a cystic lesion to establish the diagnosis, however.

Neoplastic cysts (cystadenoma or cystadenocarcinoma) must be distinguished from pseudocysts.[10] The former should be suspected when cysts are multiple, there is calcification in the cyst's wall, they occur in a patient with no previous history of pancreatitis, or they recur soon after an internal drainage operation that should have cured them. Pseudocysts should have their wall biopsied at operation to avoid this mistake.

Complications

Infection of pseudocysts is a rare but serious complication. It should be suspected when the patient develops high fever, chills, and leukocytosis. The distinction between an infected pseudocyst and a pancreatic abscess in this setting is important, although prompt drainage is necessary in both cases. Because the contents of an infected pseudocyst are liquid, however, percutaneous drainage using a catheter is often effective.[11] If surgery is performed instead, internal drainage should be done only if the anterior wall of the cyst is already firmly adherent to the posterior wall of the stomach. Then a cystgastrostomy is acceptable. In other cases the cyst should be drained externally, since an anastomosis is unlikely to heal in the face of infection. As discussed previously, abscesses always require surgical drainage.

Rupture of a pseudocyst occurs in less than 5% of cases. It presents as a sudden abdominal catastrophe with boardlike abdominal rigidity and severe pain. The cyst contents produce a chemical peritonitis similar to that caused by a perforated duodenal ulcer. The treatment is emergency surgery, extensive irrigation of the peritoneal cavity, and a drainage procedure for the pseudocyst. If the wall of the cyst is firm enough, and if the patient's condition is satisfactory, internal drainage may be performed. The wall of the cyst is usually too weak to hold sutures, however, and external drainage is required. This is a serious complication, and the mortality rate may exceed 50%.

Hemorrhage into the pseudocyst cavity or an adjacent viscus into which the cyst has eroded may present as a surgical emergency. Bleeding into the cyst may produce a rapidly enlarging, tender abdominal mass. Erosion into the stomach may be associated with hematemesis or melena. When the rate of bleeding is rapid, hemorrhagic shock is a prominent part of the clinical picture. If the bleeding has occurred more slowly, anemia may be present. If the patient's condition permits, arteriography may provide valuable information about the site of bleeding. Often, however, immediate laparotomy is necessary as a life-saving measure. The cyst should be excised along with the bleeding vessel when possible. A less satisfactory option is suture ligation of the vessel, but bleeding is more likely to recur. The splenic or gastroduodenal arteries within the cyst cavity are the most common bleeding sources. They are apparently eroded by the pancreatic enzymes in the cyst fluid.

Treatment

Pseudocysts that are larger than 5 cm and all pseudocysts that are symptomatic should be treated surgically to relieve symptoms and prevent complications. A pseudocyst arising from acute pancreatitis should be managed medically for the first 4 to 6 weeks; then operation should be performed. The waiting period allows the cyst wall to become fibrous enough to hold sutures so that an internal drainage procedure can be done safely. Waiting beyond this time increases the risk of complications. A pseudocyst that arises in a patient with chronic pancreatitis without a preceding episode of acute inflammation does not require a waiting period before surgery. Three options are available for surgical treatment: excision, external drainage, and internal drainage.

Excision is the most definitive treatment but it is technically possible in only a few cases. It is done most often for cysts in the distal body or tail of the pancreas that follow trauma. In these cases the remaining pancreas is normal, and the patient is cured by the removal of the cyst.

External drainage is used in critically ill patients or when the cyst wall is too weak to hold sutures for an anastomosis. A large-bore drainage tube (eg, 28 to 30 French) is sewn into the cyst and the other end is brought to the outside through the abdominal wall creating an external fistula. The drainage eventually stops in most patients and the tube can be pulled. If it does not, an operation may be required later to drain the fistula internally. External drainage of a pseudocyst is complicated by later recurrence of the cyst in about 20% of cases.

Internal drainage is the preferred method in most patients. The cyst is anastomosed to the stomach (cystgastrostomy), duodenum (cystduodenostomy), or to a Roux-en-Y limb of jejunum (cystjejunostomy). The interior of the cyst should be inspected for any evidence of tumor and a biopsy taken of the cyst wall. In patients who have jaundice in association with a pseudocyst, an operative cholangiogram should be performed after the cyst has been drained to confirm that the obstruction is relieved. Occasionally the bile duct will be compressed by the fibrotic pancreas. Then a biliary bypass (eg, choledochoduodenostomy) also should be done. After internal drainage, the cyst cavity shrinks and disappears within a few weeks in most cases. Patients may eat a regular diet within a week of the operation, even before the cyst has been obliterated.

Percutaneous drainage of pseudocysts has been used both as definitive nonsurgical treatment and as a temporizing measure before operation.[12] In the former instance, there appears to be an unacceptably high incidence of recurrence, similar to the situation with surgical external drainage. In the latter case, percutaneous drainage may allow surgery to be postponed so that it can be done more safely or definitively. For example, it can be used in a critically ill patient with an infected pseudocyst, or in the case of an enlarging thin-walled cyst where there may be concern about imminent rupture. Then operation can be done later when the patient is in better condition, or when the cyst wall has matured so that an internal drainage procedure is possible.

Endoscopic drainage of pseudocysts has also been reported.[13] In these cases the cysts have been situated posterior to the stomach or in the head of the pancreas adjacent to the duodenum (Fig. 7.1). The outline of the cyst is seen where it distorts the gastric or duodenal wall, and an incision is made through the bowel wall and into the cyst with electrocautery (Fig. 7.2). Internal drainage of the cysts has been achieved without surgery.

CASE PRESENTATION

> A 43-year-old alcoholic patient was evaluated for pain, nausea, vomiting, and jaundice after a bout of pancreatitis. A pseudocyst in the head of the pancreas was opacified by endoscopic cannulation (Fig. 7.1). Upper gastrointestinal endoscopy revealed extrinsic compression of the duodenum (Fig. 7.2A). Endoscopic drainage of the cyst was accomplished by cutting the duodenal wall (see Fig. 7.2B) and the cyst wall (see Fig. 7.2C). Adequate drainage by endoscopic cystduodenostomy was achieved with relief of the symptoms (see Fig. 7.2D).

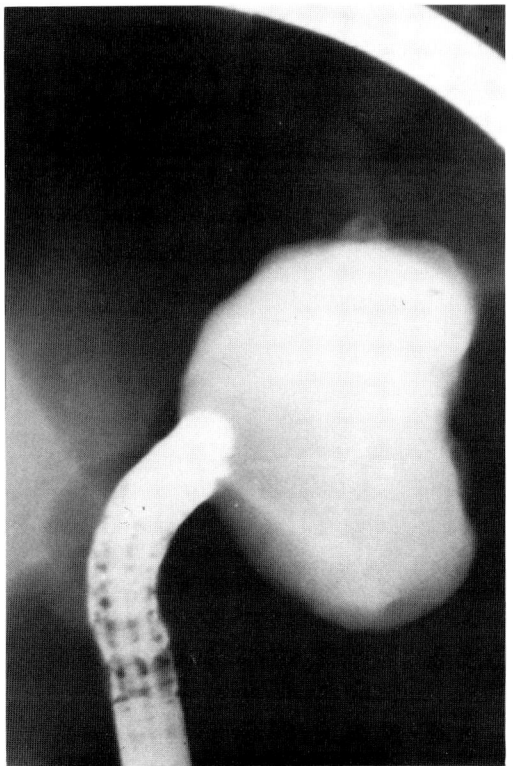

FIGURE 7.1. Pancreatic pseudocyst distorting duodenal wall and opacified by contrast injected via an endoscopically inserted catheter through the duodenal wall.

More experience with both of these techniques is required before their proper place in the management of pseudocysts is known.

Prognosis

The recurrence rate for pancreatic pseudocysts is 5% to 10% when internal drainage is performed, and about 20% with external drainage. Postoperative hemorrhage from the cyst has been reported as a rare complication, usually after cystgastrostomy.[14] The long-term outlook is influenced mainly by the underlying pancreatic inflammatory disease.

Possible outcome and management of acute pancreatitis is summarized in Table 7.1.

PANCREATIC ASCITES

Pancreatic ascites is an accumulation of free intraperitoneal fluid, the origin of which is a chronically leaking pseudocyst or a disrupted pancreatic duct. It is most

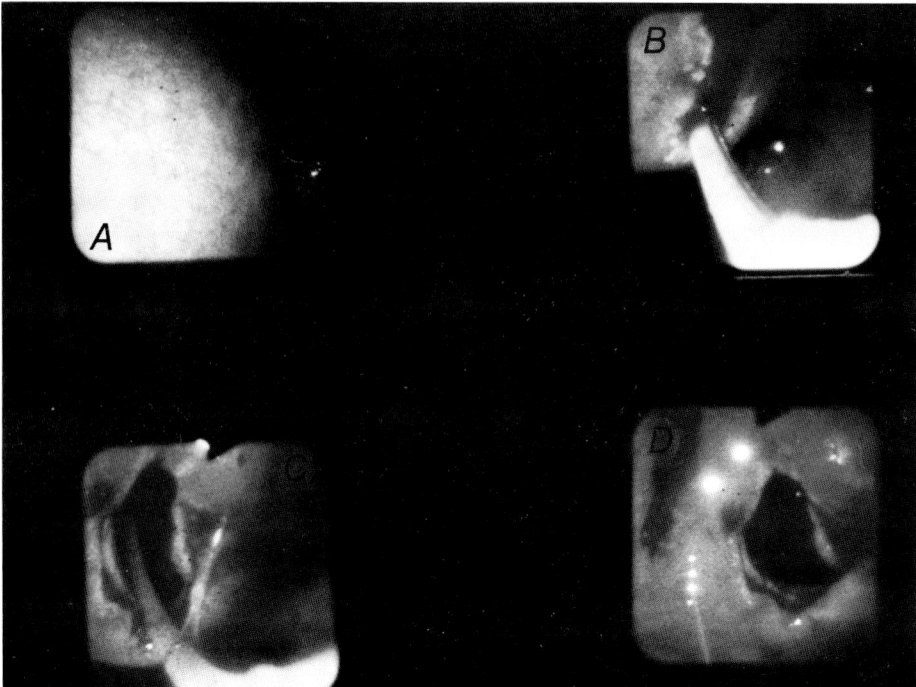

FIGURE 7-2. Endoscopic views of a pancreatic pseudocyst drained using endoscopic techniques. A. Pancreatic pseudocyst bulging into duodenum. B. Initiation of incision of duodenum. C. Completion of incision. Catheter seen entering deep into pseudocyst. D. Gaping pseudocyst-enterostomy created endoscopically (Courtesy of Dr. J. Escourroui).

TABLE 7.1. Outcome and Management of Acute Pancreatitis

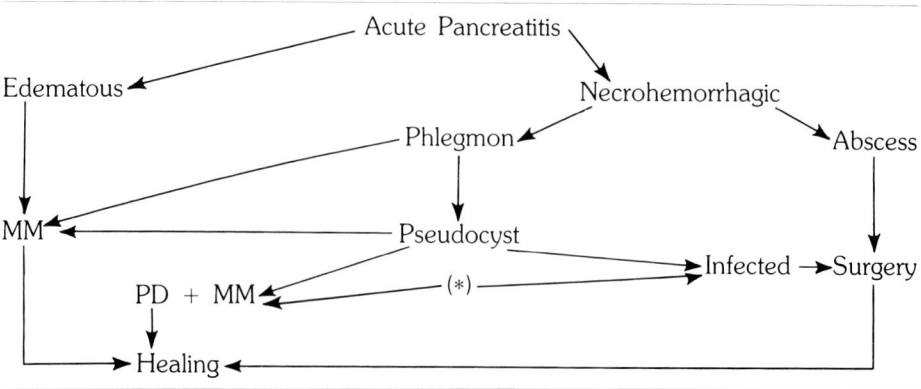

MM = Medical Management
PD = Percutaneous Drainage
* = In Some Well-defined Cases

TABLE 7.2. Characteristics of Ascitic Fluid

Disease	Protein Content (gm/dL)	White Cells	Amylase Content	Serum/Ascites Albumin Gradient
Cirrhosis	Low (≤2 g/dL)	Low (<250/mm^3)	Low	>1.1
Cirrhosis with SBP	Low	High (>250/mm^3)	Low	>1.1
Malignancy	High	Low	Low	<1.1
Pancreatic ascites	High (>3 gm/dL)	Low	High	<1.1

SBP, spontaneous bacterial peritonitis.

common in male alcoholics who have chronic pancreatitis. Occasionally it follows pancreatic trauma. The usual findings are gradually increasing abdominal girth, weight loss, and mild abdominal pain. Often there is muscle wasting and the patients appear chronically ill. The abdominal distention is often massive. Abdominal paracentesis is diagnostic: the fluid has a high total protein concentration (>3.0 g protein/dL) and the amylase concentration is always elevated above the serum level. In a recent review, the average ascitic fluid protein concentration in uninfected cirrhotic ascites was 2.0 g/dL, in infected ascites 1.6 g/dL, and in malignant ascites 1.9 g/dL.[15] Unless the patient is severely hypoalbuminemic, the ascitic fluid protein concentration in a patient with pancreatic ascites is greater than 3.0 g/dL and the gradient between serum albumin and ascitic fluid albumin is less than 1.1.

In alcoholic patients with ascites, muscle wasting, malnutrition, and hypoalbuminemia, an erroneous diagnosis of decompensated Laennec's cirrhosis is often made.[16-18] Thus, all patients with previously unrecognized ascites, particularly those with an alcoholic history, should undergo diagnostic paracentesis. The fluid should be analyzed for protein, glucose, and amylase concentrations, and cell count, differential, and bacteriologic culture also should be done (Table 7.2).

When the pancreatic fluid leak communicates directly with the peritoneal cavity, pancreatic ascites results. If the fluid leaks into the retroperitoneal space instead, it can track some distance from its origin (pleural space, mediastinum, groin) before it accumulates. About one third of patients with pancreatic ascites have pleural effusions. It is unclear why the acute rupture of a pseudocyst produces intense abdominal pain and is a surgical emergency and the chronic leakage of pancreatic fluid is much better tolerated. There is no significant peritoneal irritation and the only discomfort seems to be due to the abdominal distention.

The treatment consists of total parenteral nutrition and general correction of associated nutritional, metabolic, and immunologic abnormalities. Nothing is permitted by mouth in an effort to avoid the stimulation of pancreatic secretion. During this time the ascites may resolve in as many as 40% of cases, although it often recurs (see subsequent case presentation). The mortality rate with conservative therapy is also high (25% to 50%), however, probably as a reflection of the severely debilitated state of these patients. In most cases surgery is required to permanently eradicate the problem.

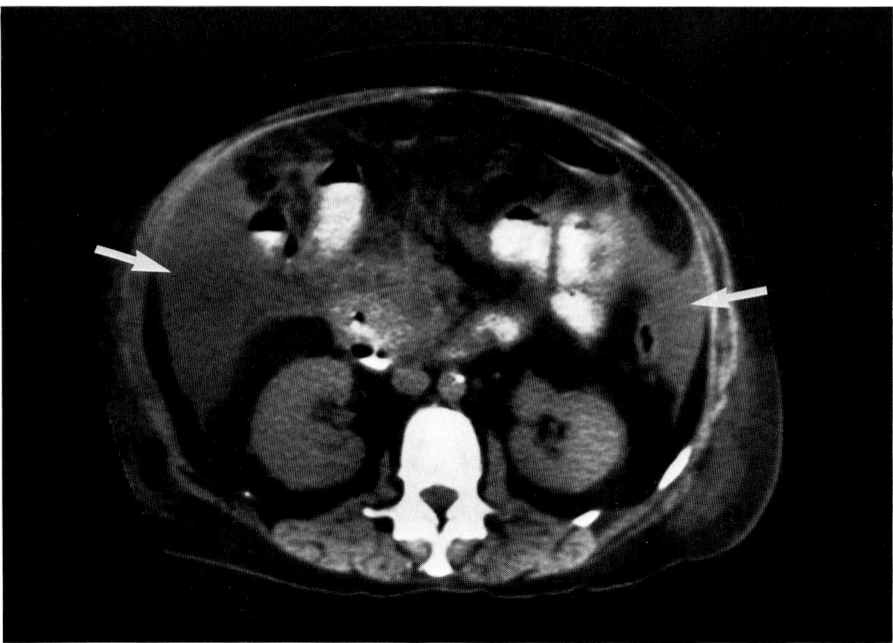

FIGURE 7.3. CT scan of the abdomen revealing a mass in the region of the head of the pancreas and ascites (arrows).

Preoperative identification of the site of leakage by ERCP has greatly simplified surgical management.[19] If the leak is in the tail of the pancreas, distal pancreatectomy is probably the best approach. If it is located elsewhere within the gland, internal drainage using a Roux-en-Y limb of jejunum is preferred. The success rate among different reports varies between 70% and 100%.

External drainage should be done only when resection or internal drainage are contraindicated for technical reasons or when the patient is critically ill. It is associated with a higher chance for recurrence (persistence) of the leak.

Others have suggested that the ascites should be removed completely to promote the apposition of intraabdominal structures to the site of the leak. Diuretics have been used as well. None of these approaches is of proven value. Experience with somatostatin, a potent inhibitor of pancreatic secretion, suggests that it may have some use in these patients.[20] Further studies are needed to be certain.

CASE PRESENTATION

A 43-year-old woman who was a known alcoholic and had previous admissions for pancreatitis was evaluated for abdominal pain and ascites with elevated amylase concentration (>1000 U/dL) in the ascitic fluid. Transverse CT scan of the pancreas revealed a mass in the region of the head of the pancreas with moderate ascites in both gutters (Fig. 7.3). The patient was treated with pain medications, parenteral nutrition, and administration

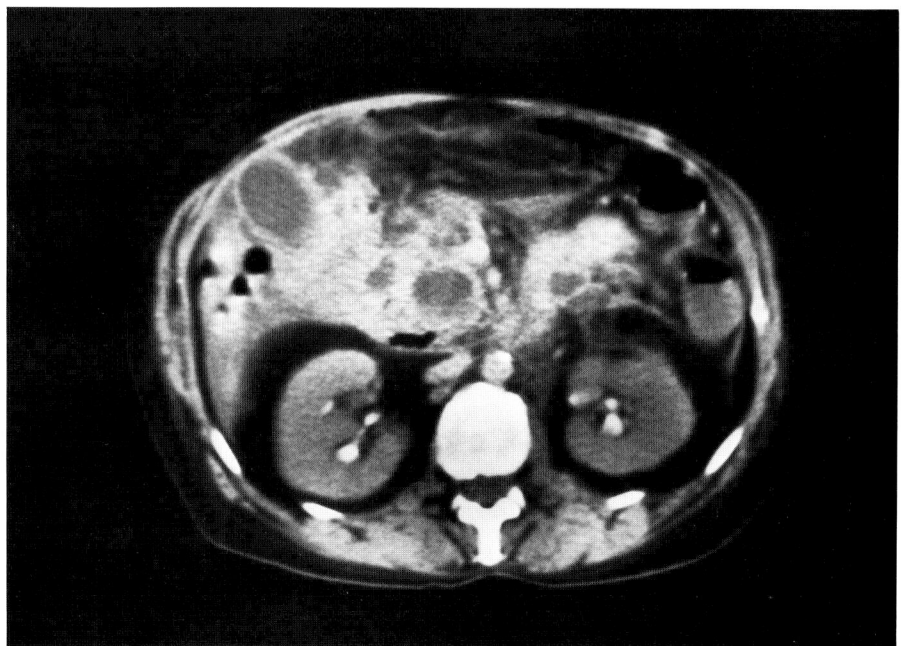

FIGURE 7.4. CT scan of the abdomen obtained 1 month later on same patient of Figure 7.3. Note reduction in the pancreatic inflammatory mass and ascites.

of a somatostatin analogue. A follow-up CT scan 1 month later revealed marked decrease in the pancreatic inflammation changes and marked decrease of ascites (Fig. 7.4).

This case is a good example of adequate response to medical therapy. Other cases develop refractory ascites and surgical treatment is ultimately necessary. In these cases a preoperative ERCP helps to identify the communication between the pancreatic duct and the peritoneal cavity.

PANCREATIC INJURY

The pancreas lies deep within the upper abdomen, in contact posteriorly with major arteries and veins and the thick paraspinal muscles and anteriorly with the intraabdominal organs. For these reasons pancreatic injury occurs only with deep penetrating wounds or blunt trauma of significant force.

Injury to the pancreas must be considered in all patients who sustain injury to the upper abdomen. However, the diagnostic approach varies with the wounding agent. With penetrating trauma almost all patients are operated on, and the diagnosis of pancreatic injury is made when the pancreas is explored.

The diagnosis of blunt pancreatic injury requires a high degree of suspicion since symptoms may be minimal or absent during the initial phase of management; this is particularly true when dealing with an isolated pancreatic injury. Days may pass before the intraabdominal accumulation of pancreatic secretions results in symptoms. For these reasons repeated abdominal examinations are mandatory. The majority of patients will ultimately develop significant epigastric pain, back pain, nausea, vomiting, and tenderness to deep palpation. Serum amylase is often normal in the immediate post trauma period, especially in patients with penetrating injuries. However, serial determinations reveal an elevated serum amylase in at least 80% of all patients with blunt pancreatic injury.[21] It is of note that an elevated level of serum amylase is not in itself a reason for surgical intervention. Corroborative evidence from physical examination, CT scan, or ultrasound is required. Diagnostic peritoneal lavage may be of particular value since many patients with serious pancreatic injury have associated visceral damage that will result in a positive lavage. The finding of an elevated amylase in the lavage fluid is also suggestive of significant pancreatic injury although a normal level does not rule out that possibility. It is important to remember that the CT scan may be inaccurate in the diagnosis of pancreatic injury. Its use should be restricted to patients in whom there is some suspicion of injury but in whom surgical intervention will be deferred unless the test is positive. There have been several reports of the use of endoscopic retrograde cholangiopancreatography (ERCP) in the diagnosis of pancreatic injury. However, in the presence of pancreatic trauma this invasive test can aggravate the damage already done. Furthermore, in the reported literature to date virtually all patients who had a diagnosis of pancreatic injury by ERCP had other indications for abdominal exploration before ERCP was performed.[22] Therefore, ERCP is of doubtful utility in the diagnosis of *acute* pancreatic injury. However, ERCP may be useful in the patient who has a pancreatic injury which presents itself with a pseudocyst or abdominal pain at a later time.

Operative management of pancreatic injury depends on its location and severity. Minor contusions and lacerations without evidence of ductal injury require only the control of hemorrhage and drainage. Deeper lacerations or crush injuries with ductal injury are best treated by distal resection of the injured gland and drainage.[23] The most difficult problem occurs when the wound is in the head of the pancreas and there is question about damage to the major pancreatic duct. If it can be ascertained easily that the duct is not injured, the treatment of wounds to the head of the pancreas is also the control of bleeding and wide drainage. When the major duct is injured, however, operative management decisions become more difficult. Pancreaticoduodenectomy is rarely done for patients with extensive injury. Lesser procedures are often preferred. One particular procedure is the drainage of the injured pancreas with diversion of pancreatic, duodenal, and gastric secretions.

Pancreatic injury is attended by a significant morbidity and mortality rate close to 20%. The majority of deaths occur from hemorrhage due to injuries to the adjacent large intraabdominal blood vessels rather than to the pancreas itself.

The most common complication of pancreatic injury is pancreatic cutaneous fistula which occurs in approximately 10% of all patients. Fistulas should initially be treated conservatively since the majority heal spontaneously. Occasionally surgery is necessary in order to achieve closure. Abdominal abscess occurs in about 5% of all patients after pancreatic injury. Another reported complication is traumatic pancreatitis. However, this is really a misnomer since elevation of serum amylase concentrations is a normal consequence of pancreatic injury. Rarely do patients develop a severe necrotizing inflammatory process in the pancreas.

References

1. Beger HG. Surgical management of necrotizing pancreatitis. In: Reber HA, ed. *The Pancreas.* Philadelphia: WB Saunders; 1989:529–549.
2. Gerzof SG, Banks PA, Robbins AH, et al. Early diagnosis of pancreatic infection by computed tomography-guided aspiration. *Gastroenterology* 1987;93:1315.
3. Block S, Maier W, Bittner R, et al. Identification of pancreas necrosis in severe acute pancreatitis: imaging procedures versus clinical staging. *Gut* 1986;27:1035.
4. Stone HH, Strom PR, Mullins RJ, et al. Pancreatic abscess management by subtotal resection and packing. *World J Surg* 1984;8:340.
5. Stricker PD, Hunt DR. Surgical aspects of pancreatic abscess. *Br J Surg* 1986;73:644.
6. Malangoni MA, Richardson SD, Shallcross JC, et al. Factors contributing to fatal outcome after treatment of pancreatic abscess. *Ann Surg* 1986;203:605.
7. Beger HG, Buchler M, Bittner R, et al. Necrosectomy and postoperative local lavage in patients with necrotizing pancreatitis: results of a prospective clinical trial. *World J Surg* 1988;12:255.
8. Crass RA, Way LW. Acute and chronic pancreatic pseudocysts are different. *Am J Surg* 1981;142:660–663.
9. Bradley EL III, Clements JL, Gonzales AC. The natural history of pancreatic pseudocysts: a unified concept of management. *Am J Surg* 1979;137:135–141.
10. Friedman AC, Lichtenstein JE, Dachman AH. Cystic neoplasms of the pancreas. *Radiology* 1983;149:45–50.
11. Gerzof SG, Willard CJ, Robins AH, et al. Percutaneous drainage of infected pancreatic pseudocysts. *Arch Surg* 1984;119:888–893.
12. Van Sonnenberg E, Casola G, Varney RR, et al. Imaging and interventional radiology for pancreatitis and its complications. *Radiol Clin North Am* 1989;27:65–72.
13. Nunez D Jr, et al. Transgastric drainage of pancreatic fluid collections. *AJR* 1985;145:815–818.
14. Stabile BE, Wilson SE, Debas HT. Reduced mortality from bleeding pseudocysts and pseudoaneurysms caused by pancreatitis. *Arch Surg* 1983;118:45–51.
15. Bar-Meier S, Lerner E, Conn HO. Analysis of ascitic fluid in cirrhosis. *Dig Dis Sci* 1979;24:136–144.
16. Broe PJ, Cameron JL. Pancreatic ascites and pancreatic pleural effusion. In: Bradley EL III, ed. *Complications of Pancreatitis.* Philadelphia: WB Saunders; 1982:245–264.
17. Maule WF, Reber HA. Diagnosis and management of pancreatic pseudocysts, pancreatic ascites, and pancreatic fistulas. In: Go VLM, Gardner JD, Brooks FP, et al, eds. *The Exocrine Pancreas: Biology, Pathobiology and Diseases:* New York, Raven Press; 1985:601–610.
18. Weaver DW, Walt AJ, Sugawa, et al. A continuing appraisal of pancreatic ascites. *Surg Gynecol Obstet* 1982;154:845–848.
19. Sankaran S, Sugawa C, Walt AJ. Value of endoscopic retrograde pancreatography in pancreatic ascites. *Surg Gynecol Obstet* 1979;148:185–192.
20. Ellison EC, Garner WL, Mekhjian HS, et al. Successful treatment of pancreatic ascites with somatostatin analog. *Gastroenterology* 1986;90:1405. Abstract.

21. Moretz JA, Campbell DP, Parker DE, et al. Significance of serum amylase level in evaluating pancreatic trauma. *Am J Surg* 1975;130:739.
22. Bozymski EM, Orlando RC, Holt JW, III. Traumatic disruption of the pancreatic duct demonstrated by endoscopic retrograde pancreatography. *J Trauma* 1981;21:244.
23. Yellin AE, Vecchione TR, Donovan AJ. Distal pancreatectomy for pancreatic trauma. *Am J Surg* 1972;124:135.

Chapter 8

Systemic Complications of Acute Pancreatitis

JAMES H. GRENDELL
DAVID A. GOLDSTEIN

Acute pancreatitis can result in derangement of a number of different organ systems leading to a severe, prolonged course and, in some patients, death.[1] Because there is no specific therapy capable of arresting or reversing the acute inflammatory process in the pancreas, much of the management of patients with acute pancreatitis depends on the early recognition and appropriate treatment of its complications (Fig. 8.1).

CARDIOVASCULAR COMPLICATIONS

In severe acute pancreatitis, a number of factors may contribute to the marked hypovolemia and hemodynamic instability frequently encountered early in the course of the disease, including exudation of plasma into the retroperitoneum and peritoneal cavity; "third-spacing" of fluid into an atonic stomach or small intestine due to a paralytic ileus; peripheral vasodilation and increased vascular permeability; hemorrhage; and vomiting. This leads to the hypotension observed in about one third of patients and may proceed to shock and multisystem organ failure. The need for massive volume replacement has been recognized as a predictor of poor outcome.

Patients with moderate-to-severe acute pancreatitis need to be monitored closely for evidence of volume depletion by frequent assessments of pulse and blood pressure (both supine and after postural change), urine output, hematocrit, and blood urea nitrogen concentration. Hypovolemia should be aggressively treated when present. Although the choice of solution is disputed, crystalloid solutions adjusted as needed to correct serum electrolyte abnormalities are effective and relatively inexpensive. Administration of albumin or other colloids to maintain plasma oncotic pressure has not been shown to be more effective than use of crystalloids in this setting and may exacerbate noncardiogenic pulmonary edema, when present.

Patients who remain hypotensive despite what appears to be adequate volume replacement require more intensive hemodynamic monitoring and assessment, with

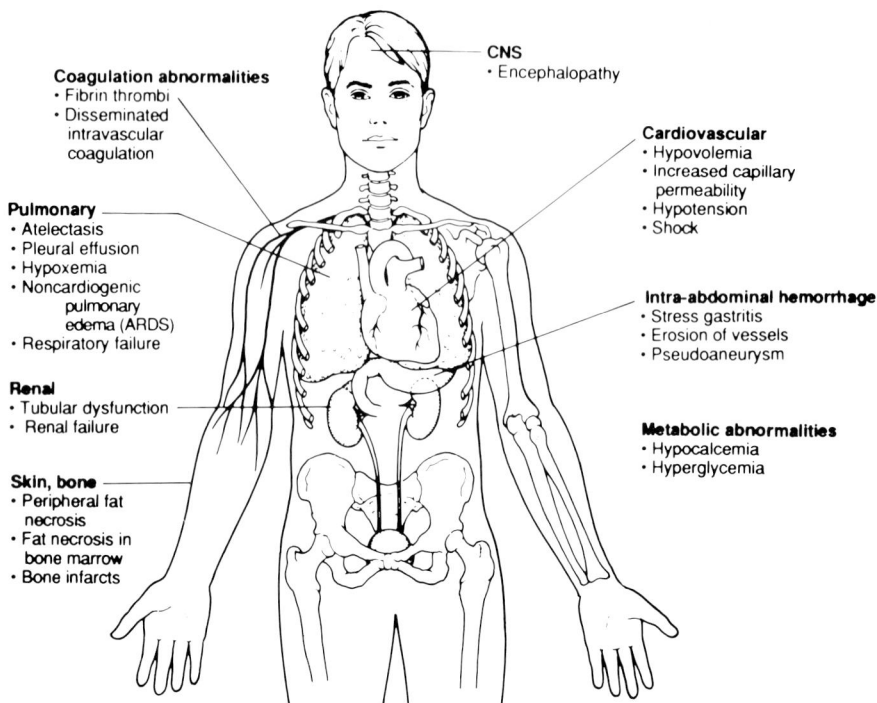

FIGURE 8.1. Major systemic complications observed in patients with acute pancreatitis.

placement of an arterial line to measure blood pressure and a pulmonary artery catheter to determine pulmonary arterial and capillary wedge pressures, cardiac index, and systemic vascular resistance. In severe acute pancreatitis these measurements may demonstrate a pattern similar to what is observed in septic shock, with hypotension resulting from a marked reduction in systemic vascular resistance despite an increased cardiac index and adequate right-sided cardiac filling pressures.[2] In this case use of a vasopressor agent such as dopamine will be required (see subsequent case presentation).

PULMONARY COMPLICATIONS

A spectrum of pulmonary complications may develop in the setting of acute pancreatitis. Nonspecific chest roentgenogram abnormalities such as basilar atelectasis and small pleural effusions are common. Arterial hypoxemia, frequently clinically "silent," has been observed in 50% or more of patients. The most serious complication, associated with substantial mortality, is development of acute respiratory failure in about 10% of patients resulting from noncardiogenic pulmonary edema (adult

SYSTEMIC COMPLICATIONS

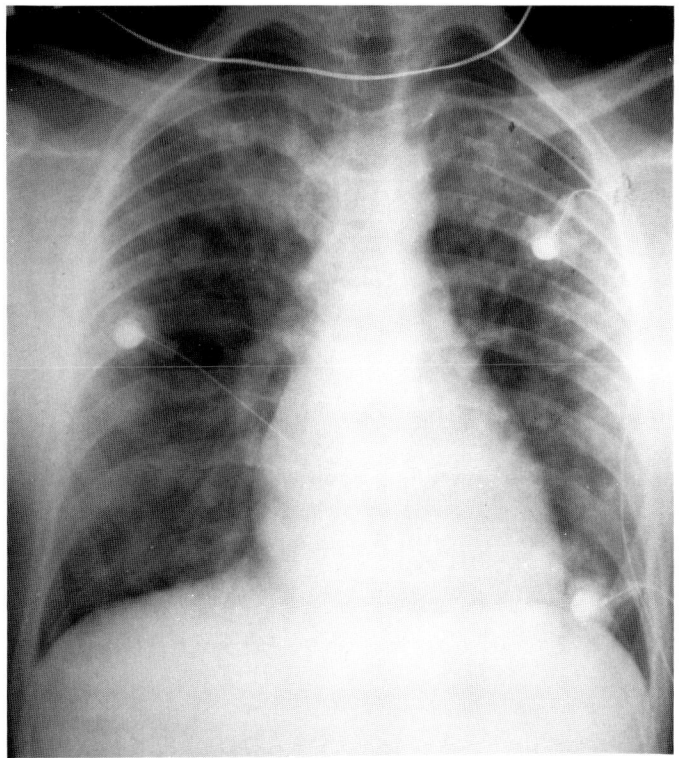

FIGURE 8.2. Chest roentgenogram showing bilateral pulmonary infiltrates in a patient with acute pancreatitis complicated by noncardiogenic pulmonary edema (adult respiratory distress syndrome) (Courtesy of P Goodman, MD).

respiratory distress syndrome [ARDS]). This is due to an increase in the permeability of the pulmonary capillary endothelium presumably caused by release of one or more toxic agents initiated by acute inflammation of the pancreas (Fig. 8.2).

The development of acute respiratory failure frequently occurs insidiously during the first week of hospitalization, in some cases in patients who on admission had normal arterial blood gas determinations and chest roentgenograms. Early signs include tachypnea and agitation, with arterial blood gas measurements indicating worsening hypoxemia and chest roentgenogram showing the progressive development of acute renal failure, which, in the setting of acute pancreatitis, carries a mortality of 50% or greater in some series.[3]

In patients with acute pancreatitis, the degree of respiratory effort, chest findings, and arterial blood gas values should be monitored closely, especially during the first few days of hospitalization. Supplemental oxygen should be provided as needed. Patients who develop acute respiratory failure will require endotracheal intubation and mechanical ventilation. Placement of a pulmonary artery catheter to help regulate volume replacement and the use of diuretics are often of great value.[4]

Acute respiratory failure may also develop later in the course of acute pancreatitis (after the first week of hospitalization) as a manifestation of sepsis, particularly the development of a pancreatic abscess. In this case appropriate antibiotic coverage and urgent surgical drainage of the abscess are required in addition to ventilatory support.[5]

RENAL COMPLICATIONS

As with pulmonary abnormalities, a spectrum of renal complications may occur in acute pancreatitis. Subclinical abnormalities in tubular function are frequently observed, characterized by an increased urinary excretion of low molecular weight proteins.[6,7] This accounts for the elevated amylase:creatinine clearance ratio found in many patients. It is not clear whether this process is related to the development of acute renal failure, which, in the setting of acute pancreatitis, carries a mortality of 50% or greater in some series.

The mechanism by which acute renal failure occurs in acute pancreatitis remains obscure. In some patients it is associated with hypotension and probably represents a form of acute tubular necrosis. Acute renal failure can occur in the absence of systemic hypotension, however. In these cases other factors may be operative, such as selective renal vasoconstriction, or direct glomerular or tubular damage produced by circulating pancreatic digestive enzymes (eg, phospholipase A_2) or by other toxic factors generated by acute inflammation of the pancreas.

The therapy of acute renal failure in this setting is similar to that for renal failure with other causes. Less severe cases can be treated by careful fluid and electrolyte management and restriction of dietary protein if the patient is eating, or provision of special essential amino acid mixtures ("renal failure" formulas) in the setting of enteral or parenteral nutrition. Severe renal failure requires dialysis either by hemodialysis or peritoneal dialysis. Because this usually occurs in the setting of acute pancreatitis with multiple complications, however, the prognosis is guarded even with adequate dialysis.

COAGULATION ABNORMALITIES

In patients and experimental animals with acute pancreatitis, intravascular fibrin thrombi are frequently present in the pancreas and peripancreatic fat as well as in other organs such as the kidney, lung, and adrenal gland.[8,9] In addition, early in the course of the disease some patients will demonstrate evidence of disseminated intravascular coagulation characterized by falling platelet counts and plasma fibrinogen concentrations and increasing levels of products of fibrin degradation. The basis of these abnormalities remains uncertain but trypsin released from the inflamed pancreas is a potential major factor. Later in the course of acute pancreatitis, platelet counts and plasma fibrinogen levels may rise above the normal range.

Neither clinical nor experimental studies have clarified whether the coagulation abnormalities and intravascular thrombosis observed in acute pancreatitis are significant contributors of the damage produced in the pancreas and other organs, or whether these are merely reflective of tissue injury. Limited clinical experience with heparin administration has not demonstrated it to be beneficial and suggests the possibility of an increased risk of hemorrhage. No specific therapy directed at the coagulation system in acute pancreatitis appears indicated, apart from correcting vitamin K deficiency, when present.

Hemorrhage

Several clincal series have demonstrated a 5% to 10% incidence of significant upper gastrointestinal bleeding in the setting of acute pancreatitis, typically caused by stress ulcers, peptic ulcers, or esophageal or gastric varices. Bleeding from stress ulcers has been reported in about 15% of patients with severe acute pancreatitis or pancreatic abscesses. Thus, patients with severe acute pancreatitis, especially those with multiple risk factors for bleeding from stress gastritis (eg, respiratory or renal failure, hypotension, sepsis) should receive appropriate prophylaxis against this problem by means of antacid titration or administration of an H_2-antagonist or sucralfate. Once significant upper gastrointestinal bleeding has occurred, endoscopy should be performed to identify the source. Because patients with severe acute pancreatitis are frequently not good candidates for operative intervention to control bleeding, when feasible, endoscopic coagulation or sclerosing methods or angiographic approaches to controlling bleeding, should be employed first.

An additional potentially lethal cause of hemorrhage in acute pancreatitis is disruption of a major vessel by the inflammatory process. This may lead either to massive intraabdominal hemorrhage or to bleeding into the gastrointestinal tract by way of the pancreatic duct. Angiography is the best means of identifying the source of bleeding and provides a means of controlling this type of bleeding using angiographic embolization of the bleeding vessel (Fig. 8.3). If this is unsuccessful, operative management is necessary but carries a high mortality.

METABOLIC ABNORMALITIES

Acute pancreatitis can result in a variety of metabolic abnormalities. In general, the more severe the attack, the more likely these will occur.[10]

Hypocalcemia

Serum calcium concentrations frequently are decreased in acute pancreatitis with a marked decrease indicative of a worse prognosis.[11] There are a number of factors that have been proposed to contribute to the development of hypocalcemia, including hypoalbuminemia, hypomagnesemia, sequestration of calcium in regions of fat necrosis, reduction in secretion of parathyroid hormone or its increased destruction, and impaired mobilization of calcium from bone in response to parathyroid hormone.[12] Although a decrease in total serum calcium concentration of the facial muscle

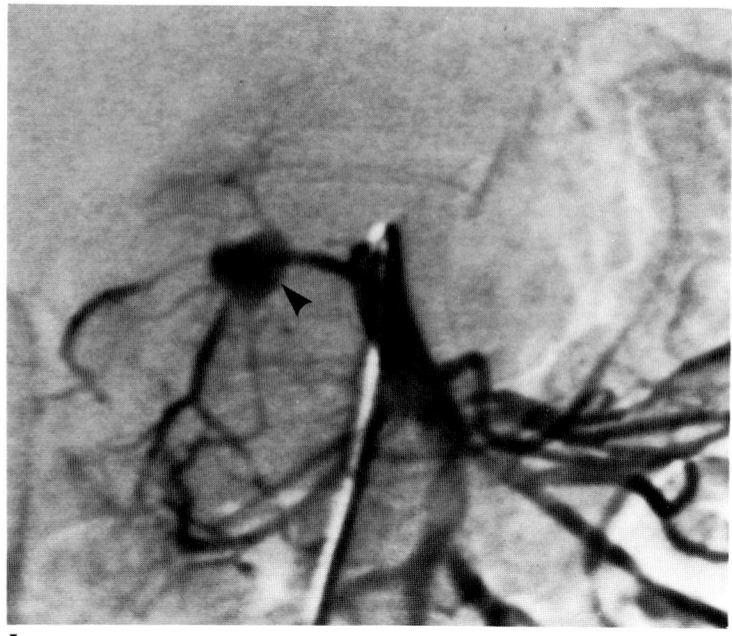

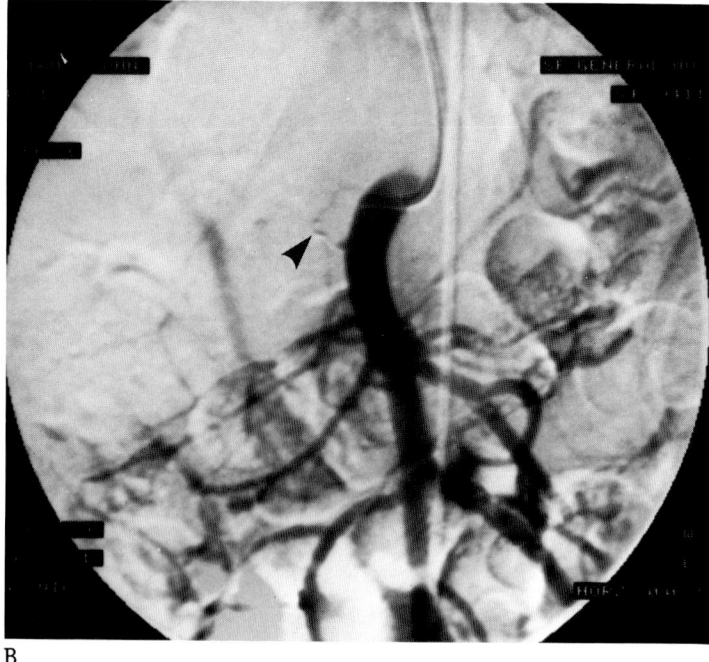

FIGURE 8.3. A: Mesenteric angiography demonstrating bleeding from a pseudoaneurysm (arrow) in a patient with acute pancreatitis. B: Successful control of bleeding in the same patient by means of angiographic embolization of the bleeding vessel with a metal coil (arrow) (Courtesy of RB Jeffrey, Jr, MD).

(Chvostek's sign) is frequently observed, however, this does not necessarily reflect a reduction in ionized calcium in plasma. Only rarely does clinically significant hypocalcemia occur as indicated by signs of tetanic contractions or prolongation of the QT interval on electrocardiography. Thus, hypocalcemia in the setting of acute pancreatitis requires urgent correction only if it is clinically significant. The serum calcium concentration should be corrected for alteration in the serum albumin. The difference in albumin concentration from a reference point of 4.0 g/dL should be multiplied by a factor of 0.8 and added or subtracted from the given value of calcium (eg, a serum of 6.5 mg/dL in the presence of an albumin of 2.5 g/dL should be altered in the following manner: $4.0 - 2.5 = 1.5 \times 0.8 = 1.2$; $6.5 + 1.2 = 7.7$; therefore the corrected serum calcium is 7.7 mg/dL.

In addition we recommend adding 10 mL ampule of 10% calcium gluconate (90 mg or 4.5 mEq of calcium) per liter of intravenous fluid if the serum calcium level (corrected for serum albumin concentration) is less than 7 mg/dL. Continue this infusion until the serum calcium reaches a range of 8.0 to 7.5 mg/dL. Hypokalemia should be corrected before intravenous administration of calcium to prevent potentially dangerous cardiac arrhythmias. Hypomagnesemia, if present, should also be corrected to enhance the effectiveness of calcium administration.

Hyperglycemia

Hyperglycemia commonly occurs early in the course of acute pancreatitis. It appears to be due to an excess of circulating glucagon with variable serum levels of insulin. Generally this is observed in the absence of ketoacidosis (except in alcoholic ketoacidosis; see subsequent sections) or severe glycosuria and does not require insulin therapy because blood sugar levels typically return to normal over several days time. Insulin administration may produce hypoglycemia, given the difficulty in determining an appropriate dose in such a highly unstable metabolic state. Ketoacidosis (except when caused by alcohol) or marked glycosuria should be treated by cautious administration of small doses of regular insulin.

Metabolic Acidosis

Patients with severe acute pancreatitis may demonstrate evidence of a metabolic acidosis on determination of serum electrolyte concentrations and arterial blood gas measurement.[13] This is usually a *lactic acidosis* caused by hypoperfusion or respiratory insufficiency. Some alcoholic patients who have not been eating regularly may present with acute pancreatitis and *alcoholic ketoacidosis*. These patients may have a large anion gap but usually only a slight-to-moderate increase in serum lactate concentration. They can be differentiated from patients with diabetic ketoacidosis by their relatively low blood fructose concentration (<300 mg/dL) and from both diabetic ketoacidosis and lactic acidosis by the disproportionate increase of β-hydroxybutyrate relative to lactate in blood (0.2:1; normal, 1:1).

Treatment of lactic acidosis requires optimizing perfusion with volume replacement and improving inadequate oxygenation. If renal failure is present, hemodialysis may be required to correct lactic acidosis. Administration of intravenous bicarbonate may transiently improve the serum bicarbonate concentration and pH, but has little effect on outcome. Alcoholic ketoacidosis can be corrected by administration of intravenous glucose. Thiamine should also be given in this setting to prevent deficiency.

FAT NECROSIS

In addition to the fat necrosis commonly observed in peripancreatic fat in the retroperitoneum and omental fat in the peritoneal cavity, distant fat necrosis may occur. This typically results in painful subcutaneous nodules, arthritis or synovitis, or bony lesions caused by necrosis of fat in the bone marrow or bone infarcts (Fig. 8.4). No specific therapy is available, and lesions typically subside with resolution of acute pancreatitis.

ENCEPHALOPATHY

A variety of neuropsychiatric symptoms and signs has been reported in the setting of acute pancreatitis. Petechial hemorrhages and demyelinization have been found in brain tissue of patients dying of this disease. It has been postulated that increased levels of lipase in cerebrospinal fluid may play a role in this process. The neuropsychiatric abnormalities reported in this setting do not fit into any well-defined syndrome, however, and probably manifest the effects of hypotension, hypoxemia, electrolyte abnormalities, analgesia, alcohol withdrawal, and other severe physiologic stresses inflicted on the central nervous systems of patients with severe acute pancreatitis.

Concomitant medical problems such as acute pancreatitis with a likelihood and severity of alcohol withdrawal symptoms may occur in patients with a history of recent heavy alcohol use and evidence of agitation, confusion, or hallucinations (auditory, visual, or tactile). They should be treated for presumed alcohol withdrawal and should be monitored carefully.

CASE PRESENTATION

> A 41-year-old man has abdominal pain of 3 days duration. He has been drinking heavily for the previous 3 weeks. Before more history can be obtained, the patient suffers a cardiorespiratory arrest. He is intubated and cardioverted from ventricular fibrillation to ventricular tachycardia. After resuscitative measures, including lidocaine, epinephrine, and magnesium sulfate, the patient is transferred to the medical intensive care unit on dopamine with a blood pressure of 128 mm Hg systolic, pulse of 100 beats/minute, temperature of 98°F, and a respiratory rate controlled by a ventilator at 20/minute. Physical examination reveals a stuporous man who moves all of his extremities spontaneously and is responsive to verbal and tactile stimuli.

SYSTEMIC COMPLICATIONS

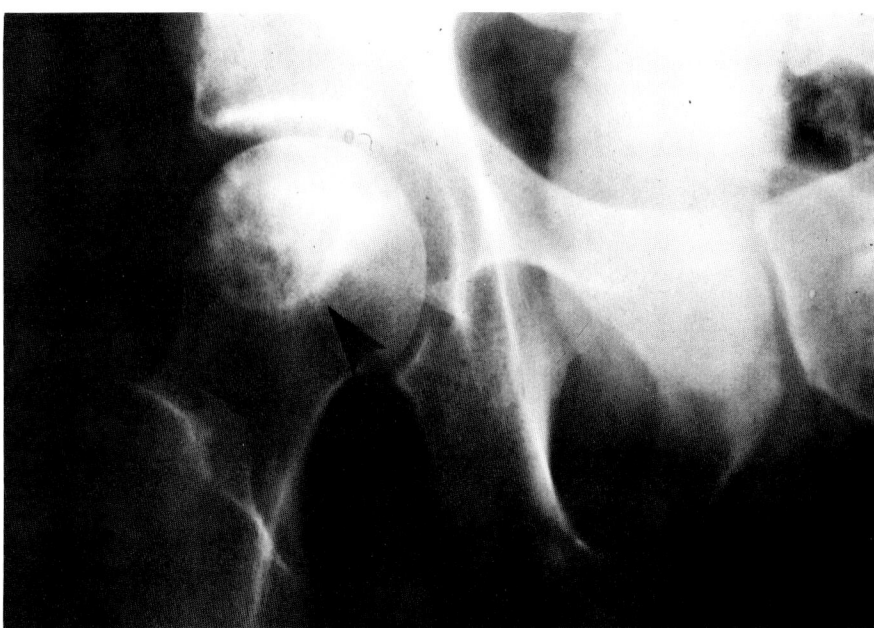

FIGURE 8.4. Roentgenogram of the head of the right femur demonstrating a bone infarct (arrow) due to fat necrosis of the marrow in a patient with acute pancreatitis (Courtesy of JE Valenzuela, MD).

There are bibasilar rales and decreased bowel sounds diffusely over the abdomen.

Laboratory data included the following: serum sodium 136; potassium 1.7; chloride 101; bicarbonate 9 mEq/L; calcium 6.7; phosphorous 1.09; magnesium 3.2; glucose 1085; blood urea nitrogen 35; creatinine 2.7 mg/dL; albumin 2.4 g/dL; white blood cell 5900/mL (30 segs, 50 bands, 11 lymphs, 9 monos); hematocrit 44%; pH 7.13; pO_2 256; pCO_2 29 mm Hg (FI O_2 100%); urine sodium 71 mEq/L; serum ketones 1:4; lipase 2186; amylase 189 U/dL; SGOT (AST) 33 IU/L; LDH 151 IU/L; lactate 1.0 mEq/L.

This patient has many of the metabolic complications of acute and severe pancreatitis. These include ketoacidosis, hypokalemia, hypophosphatemia, hypocalcemia, presumed hypomagnesemia, and acute renal failure.

It is likely that dehydration and intravascular volume depletion developed from a variety of factors. These include poor oral intake; vomiting; third space accumulation of fluids associated with the edematous pancreas, local inflammation, and resultant paralytic ileus; and osmotic diuresis secondary to the hyperglycemia. Note that the apparent normal sodium concentration is misleading. The marked elevation of serum glucose leads to a shift of water from the intracellular space to the vascular compartment, thereby diluting the serum sodium level. If a correction for this phenomenon, for example, $1.6 \times 10\%$ (serum glucose $-$ 100) is made, a serum sodium concentration of 152 mEq/1 (ie, 136 + 16) is derived. Because of the dehydrated state, the hematocrit of 44 is also falsely within the normal range, thereby masking an anemia.

Diabetic ketoacidosis is a rare complication of pancreatitis, even when the condition is hemorrhagic and not merely edematous. Alcoholic ketosis should be considered as an alternative diagnosis since it can occur in individuals who imbibe alcohol to excess. Ketosis can also occur because of prolonged fasting. Such acidosis rarely leads to serum bicarbonate concentrations of ≦16 mEq/L and more often occurs in females with excess fat stores. This ketoacid does not react with usual reagents and would be an unlikely etiologic agent in this case, in which there are ample ketone bodies identified in the serum. The patient was given magnesium sulfate at the time of the cardiorespiratory arrest. This accounts for the elevated serum magnesium. Before arrest the level should have been low because of deposition in local areas of inflammation; decreased cell catabolism; decreased oral intake and vomiting; increased renal excretion due to alcohol and the osmotic diuresis due to hyperglycemia; and decreased tubular reabsorption of magnesium associated with hyperaldosterone. The syndrome of magnesium depletion leads to hypocalcemia due to impaired secretion of parathyroid hormone (PTH) and resistance at target organs (eg, bone) to the action of PTH; cardiac arrhythmias, muscle weakness, and neuromuscular irritability.

It is known that acute renal failure can complicate acute hemorrhagic pancreatitis. The mechanism of this phenomenon is not well understood. It may accompany severe hypotension, but acute renal failure has been reported to complicate even mild pancreatitis in the absence of hypotension. Renal vasoconstriction may be causative and due to a reaction to the liberated pancreatic enzymes. These enzymes can actually damage tubular cells. Note that it is not possible to estimate the glomerular filtration rate with any degree of prognostic confidence from the single serum creatinine measurement of 2.7 mg/dL in this patient. There may be complete renal shutdown with only a moderate increase in serum creatinine since more time is necessary for a steady state to develop. Although the serum level of creatinine in this case probably represents intrinsic renal dysfunction, similar elevations can occur in severe ketosis when the ketoacidosis interferes with the colorimetric analysis of creatinine.

This patient requires aggressive management. The state of hydration as well as the electrolyte abnormalities forces the physician to address several issues simultaneously. The assessment of renal function is crucial. If the elevated urine sodium was determined before any fluid resuscitation, acute tubular necrosis would be suggested, requiring more caution. If renal shutdown had already occurred, the administration of potassium, phosphorus, and magnesium should be tempered.

This patient should be admitted to the medical intensive care unit where a balloon-tipped, flow-directed pulmonary artery catheter can be inserted to dynamically monitor hemodynamic status. This is indicated when patients with acute pancreatitis are in shock or require large volumes of fluid. The initial intravenous fluid used in this case should be normal saline. Although this option would not be as effective in alleviation of the hyperosmolar state (ie, 347 mOsm), volume and consequent maintenance of blood pressure is of primary importance. Fluid can be administered at a rate of 250 ml/h or as the Swan-Ganz data permits. Hypotonic solutions can be administered once the blood pressure is stabilized. Dextrose can be added to the infusion when serum glucose reaches 250 mg/dL.

Insulin will be an important tool in therapy. Low dose therapy should be employed. Since this patient acquired diabetes from pancreatic damage his requirements will probably be at the low end of the range, that is, loading dose of 10 to 20 units of regular insulin followed by 5 to 12 units per hour. Regular insulin should be employed when the blood glucose level reaches 250 mg/dL, and the rate of insulin infusion should fall to 1 to 4 U/h.

Renal function should be monitored carefully. A fractional excretion of sodium be determined:

$$\frac{U_{NA}}{P_{ma}} \times \frac{P_{cr}}{U_{cr}} \times 100 = FE_{na}(\%)$$

U_{na} = Urine sodium concentration (mEq/mL)
P_{na} = Plasma sodium concentration (mEq/mL)
P_{na} = Plasma creatinine concentration (mEq/mL)
U_{cr} = Urine creatinine concentration (mEq/mL)

In acute renal failure the FE_{na} is usually greater than 1% whereas in prerenal azotemia it is usually less than 1%. If this patient is in acute renal failure the replacement of electrolytes should be done as follows:

1. Potassium—the average potassium requirements in diabetic ketoacidosis range from 200 to 350 mEq during the first 24 hours. In these patients the needs will likely exceed 350 mEq. Initial therapy can begin at 20 to 40 mEq/h until the electrocardiogram has normalized and the blood level has reached less critical values >3.0 mEq/L.
2. Phosphorus—intravenous phosphorus can be administered as the inorganic salt with sodium or potassium at a rate of 2.5 to 5.0 mg/kg over 6 hours. Further therapy should be assessed only after a serum phosphorus level is obtained. Note that if potassium phosphate is used, the previous potassium recommendations need to be adjusted.
3. Magnesium—no further treatment should be given, but the level should be monitored. If profound hypomagnesemia (<1.0 mEq/L) is present, magnesium sulfate, 1 to 2 mg (8 to 16 mEq) can be administered over 20 minutes.

References

1. Pitchumoni CS, Agarwal N, Jain KN. Systemic complications in acute pancreatitis. *Am J Gastroenterol* 1988;83:597–606.
2. Beger HG, Bittner R, Buchler M, et al. Hemodynamic data pattern in patients with acute pancreatitis. *Gastroenterology* 1986;90:74–79.
3. Renner IG, Savage WT, Pantoja JL, Renner VJ. Death due to acute pancreatitis: a retrospective analysis of 405 autopsy cases. *Dig Dis Sci* 1985;30:1005–1018.
4. Basran GS, Ramasubramanian R, Verma R. Intrathoracic complications of acute pancreatitis. *Br J Dis Chest* 1987;81:326–331.
5. Lankisch PG, Rahlf G, Koop H. Pulmonary complications in fatal acute hemorrhagic pancreatitis. *Dig Dis Sci* 1983;28:111–116.
6. Mock DM, Grendell JH, Cello J, et al. Pancreatitis and alcoholism disorder the renal tubule and impair reclamation of some low molecular weight proteins. *Gastroenterology* 1987;92:161–170.

7. Meier PB, Levitt MD. Urine protein excretion in acute pancreatitis. *J Lab Clin Med* 1986; 108:628–634.
8. Lasson A, Ohlsson K. Disseminated intravascular coagulation and antiprotease activity in acute human pancreatitis. *Scand J Gastroenterol* 1986;21(suppl 126):35–39.
9. Lasson A, Ohlsson K. Consumptive coagulopathy, fibrinolysis and protease–antiprotease interactions during acute human pancreatitis. *Thromb Res* 1986;41:167–183.
10. Banks PA. Metabolic complications of pancreatitis. In Bradley EL, ed. *Complications of Pancreatitis: Medical and Surgical Management.* Philadelphia: W.B. Saunders; 1982:176–202.
11. Weir GC, Lesser PB, Drop LJ, et al. The hypocalcemia of acute pancreatitis. *Ann Intern Med* 1975;83:185–189.
12. Allan BF, Imrie CW. Serum ionized calcium in acute pancreatitis. *Br J Surg* 1977; 64:665–668.
13. Drew SI, Joffe B, Vinik A, et al. The first 24 hours of acute pancreatitis. Changes in biochemical homeostasis in patients with pancreatitis compared with those in control subjects undergoing stress for reasons other than pancreatitis. *Am J Med* 1978;64:795–803.

Chapter 9
Chronic Pancreatitis

ANDRÉ RIBET
JACQUES MOREAU
JORGE E. VALENZUELA

EPIDEMIOLOGY

Based on post mortem findings, chronic pancreatitis has a higher incidence than appreciated when diagnosed clinically and its occurrence varies in different areas of the world. Autopsy diagnosis must be accepted with caution, however, since in some instances it may be difficult to differentiate minor inflammatory changes such as fibrosis, duct abnormalities, and atrophy that occur as a consequence of aging without episodes of pain from those resulting from chronic inflammation. In spite of this reservation, it seems that the incidence of chronic pancreatitis is increasing. For instance, the incidence of chronic alcoholic pancreatitis rose in Denmark from 6.9 to 10 per 100,000 from 1970 to 1979. Similar trends are observed worldwide.[1] Obviously this may correspond to improvement in diagnostic tests. There also seems to be a true higher incidence of pancreatitis associated with malnutrition in certain tropical areas of Asia (Southern India) or Africa (Nigeria), whereas pancreatitis associated with chronic alcoholism continues to rise in some countries of Europe, the United States, Brazil, South Africa, and more recently in Japan. There seems to be some geographic variations in the clinical presentation, that is, chronic pancreatitis in the United States appears to occur mainly in chronic alcoholics with a dilated main duct but ductal obstruction is rare; in Britain alcoholic pancreatitis is less common and ductal strictures are found more often.[2] Calcifications appear to be more common in alcoholic pancreatitis compared with nonalcoholic pancreatitis in the United States and Japan, whereas no differences are observed among these groups in Europe.[3-5] These differences are probably related to the time of diagnosis of chronic pancreatitis and it seems more likely that it is one disease with protean manifestations.

Morphologically chronic pancreatitis is characterized by sclerosis, destruction and permanent loss of the pancreatic parenchyma, minimal to marked dilation of the ductal system, a variable degree of inflammatory reaction, and focal necrosis. These changes are usually progressive and irreversible. A distinct form, obstructive chronic pancreatitis, is characterized by dilation of the ductal system proximal to the occlusion of one of the major ducts, however, and these changes may be reversible when the obstruction is removed.

CLINICAL MANIFESTATIONS

Recurrent and persistent abdominal pain is one of the most frequent and earliest symptoms. It is commonly associated with weight loss; steatorrhea and diabetes occur at a later stage.

Abdominal Pain

Abdominal pain is the most common symptom, observed in 60% to 90% of patients. The proportion of patients without abdominal pain varies and seems to be affected by the selection criteria. Painful forms of pancreatitis are more common among surgical series, whereas in as many as 30% of patients with chronic pancreatitis diagnosed when diabetes was the main reason for consultation, abdominal pain was remarkably absent. Truly asymptomatic cases of chronic pancreatitis are not likely to be diagnosed. Nausea and vomiting are frequent and usually do not relieve the pain. Some patients notice some improvement in the jack-knife position. In most cases the pain is not alleviated by antacids and appears to get worse after food intake, particularly with heavy meals and alcohol ingestion.

The duration of the pain varies from a few hours to several days, and in a minority of patients it appears to become constant. Long-term studies of about 20 years on a large number of patients, revealed that about 80% of patients experience some spontaneous relief over time, as pancreatic dysfunction and calcifications become more evident. This occurs in a median period of 4.5 years after onset of the disease. The range may extend to almost 2 decades, however.[6] Although most authors have had similar experiences, the practical value of this observation in the management of the individual patient with pancreatitis remains uncertain. Although it is frequently alluded to, the association between continuous alcohol ingestion and pain in chronic pancreatitis is not clear. First, abstinence is not always total. Second, although some groups report better success after surgery in abstinents,[6,7] others have noticed no influence of continuous drinking on the postoperative outcome.[8] Third, disappearance of pain has been observed in chronic alcoholics who continue to drink, perhaps because of progressive destruction of the pancreatic parenchyma.[6]

The mechanisms for pain in chronic pancreatitis are not completely understood.[9] In the presence of pseudocysts, it is attractive to attribute the pain to the pseudocyst, and most patients appear to experience pain relief after drainage of the pseudocyst. Another common belief associates pain with pancreatic duct hypertension and distention. Abnormalities of the ductal system have been demonstrated by endoscopic retrograde pancreatography (ERP) and they are frequently considered in the decision to intervene surgically. There is no solid evidence that directly correlates dilation and abnormalities of the pancreatic ductal system and the severity of pain, however. Similarly, no positive correlation has been demonstrated between reduction in pancreatic tissue pressure as measured preoperatively and long-term pain relief after surgery.[10] Bockman et al observed that nerves are maintained within the pancreas as the parenchyma degenerates, and that these nerves increase in diameter with inflammatory reaction and ultrastructural damage in the perineurium. These authors postulated that the effect of the absence of perineurium on sensory nerves may be related to pain in chronic pancreatitis.[11]

In a few patients pain may be due to biliary stenosis caused by pancreatic fibrosis and compression of the intrapancreatic portion of the common bile duct.

Weight Loss

Whatever the mechanism, abdominal pain appears to be partially responsible for the weight loss observed as patients limit their food intake. Weight loss is a common sign of chronic pancreatitis and is often accompanied by some degree of emaciation and muscle wasting without demonstrable steatorrhea and diabetes.

Steatorrhea and Malabsorption

Steatorrhea is always considered a late sign of chronic pancreatitis since a decrease of more than 90% secretion of lipolytic enzymes is necessary before steatorrhea occurs. In malnourished and alcoholic patients, the effects of these factors on the intestinal absorptive capacity and regulatory mechanisms of intestinal function may play contributory roles.

In addition to affecting fat and protein absorption, impaired exocrine pancreatic secretion causes deficiencies of liposoluble vitamins such as vitamin A (night blindness), vitamin D (osteomalacia), vitamin E (neurologic abnormalities), vitamin K (bleeding diatheses), and vitamin B12 (macrocytosis and peripheral neuropathy). Vitamin B12 requires proteolytic enzymes to hydrolyze its binding to R factor.

Essential fatty acid deficiency also may occur. The full spectrum of clinical consequences of this deficiency is not entirely known, although dermatitis and alopecia may occur. Essential fatty acids are precursors of compounds such as prostanoids and leukotrienes and their deficiency could affect multiple cellular mechanisms. In the majority of patients (>90%) with chronic pancreatitis, exocrine pancreatic insufficiency gradually gets worse, particularly when excessive alcohol ingestion is continued. There are patients with chronic pancreatitis and moderate pancreatic secretory insufficiency who show improvement of pancreatic function after alcohol abstinence or a drainage procedure of the pancreatic duct system, however.[12] Early obstruction of the pancreatic duct may account for this favorable course. This situation may be suspected when, in the absence of an acute episode, serum pancreatic enzymes remain elevated in the patient with known chronic pancreatitis. ERP usually confirms the ductal obstruction and is also helpful to rule out a pancreatic duct tumor.

Diabetes

The exact prevalence of diabetes mellitus in chronic pancreatitis is between 30% and 70%. It is difficult to compare different studies because some clinical series include all patients with disturbances in glycoregulation, whereas others refer to symptomatic diabetes only. There is a consensus, however, that there is a close relationship between progression of the disease, increase in pancreatic calcification, and exocrine and endocrine dysfunction. Diabetes results from destruction and fibrosis of the islets cells and is aggravated during acute episodes, possibly by degradation of proinsulin and insulin by increased circulating proteases. Thus, in patients with chronic pancreatitis observed for longer than 5 years, glucose intolerance is relatively common. Ketoacidosis, retinopathy, neuropathy, and nephropathy are relatively rare, however. In chronic alcoholics, the development of cirrhosis seems to facilitate the occurrence of diabetes.

PHYSICAL EXAMINATION

In general, there is a remarkable paucity of physical findings in comparison with the severity of abdominal pain; there may be some weight loss, emaciation, and muscle wasting. The presence of a palpable mass in the midabdomen suggests a pseudocyst or a phlegmon. In a minority of chronic alcoholics, signs of chronic liver disease such as hepatomegaly, telangectasias, splenomegaly, and ascites may be found.

A summary of the symptoms and signs that may be found in chronic pancreatitis is illustrated in Figure 9.1.

COMPLICATIONS OF CHRONIC PANCREATITIS

Other symptoms of chronic pancreatitis usually result from recurrent bouts of acute pancreatitis.

Episodes of Acute Pancreatitis

About one third of patients with chronic alcoholic pancreatitis present for the first time with attacks of acute pancreatitis. Alcoholic acute pancreatitis has clinical features similar to acute episodes of pancreatitis from other causes. The severity varies from mild to severe, with an overall mortality of about 10%. Acute episodes recur, and perhaps because of the progressive destruction of the gland, their clinical course tends to become more benign and respond better to medical treatment.

Pseudocysts

In addition to congenital, parasitic, and cystic tumors, two types of pseudocysts can occur in chronic pancreatitis.

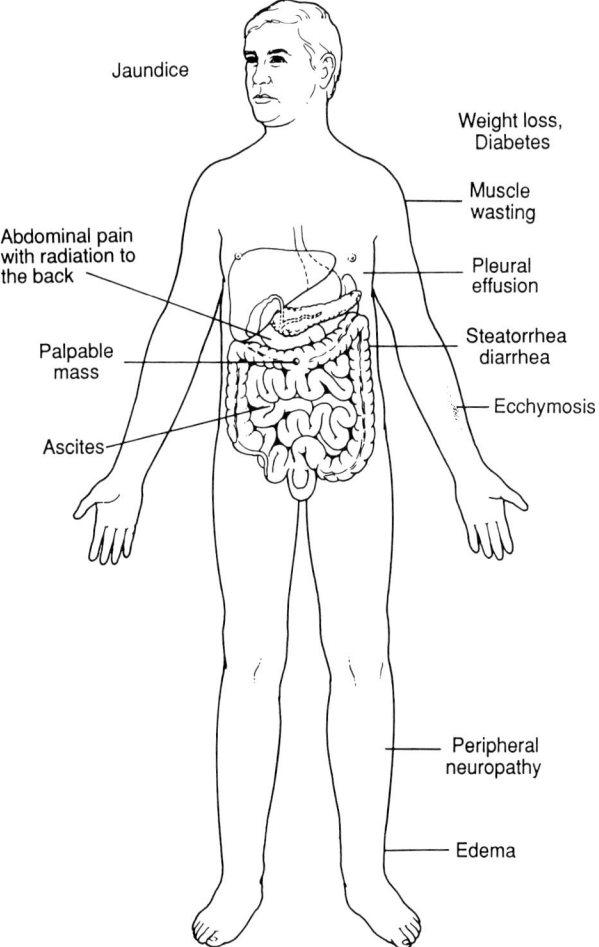

FIGURE 9.1. Possible findings in chronic pancreatitis.

Necrotic Pseudocysts (Post Acute Pancreatitis)

Some pseudocysts occur more often after acute attacks and appear to result from acute necrosis and inflammation with rupture into the peripancreatic spaces and extravasation of pancreatic juice. They occur in about one third of acute attacks of chronic pancreatitis. These "necrotic" pseudocysts are more frequently located in the body and tail of the pancreas. They may be partly extrapancreatic and after a maturation time of 4 to 6 weeks they are contained by a fibrous wall of variable thickness. Spontaneous resolution has been observed in about 10% of cases.[13,14] These pseudocysts, like others, cause mechanical complications such as obstruction of the biliary tree and obstruction of the gastroduodenal tract, and may become infected and cause gastrointestinal hemorrhage. In alcoholics the overall mortality rate is about 5%, lower than the mortality observed in necrotic pseudocysts associated with biliary pancreatitis.

Retention Pseudocysts (Chronic)

Retention pseudocysts occur without apparent relation to an acute episode of pancreatitis. They are frequently multiple; are caused by dilation of the pancreatic ducts distal to calculi, plugs, or strictures; and seem to result from ductal obstruction or "retention." The smaller cysts are all within the pancreas, and ductal epithelium can be recognized in some areas of the cyst wall. These cysts are more frequently found in the head of the pancreas (70%) and may be partly contained within the gland, but sometimes extend to more distant sites. They can be asymptomatic or cause signs and symptoms of extrinsic compression of the gut, such as gastric outlet obstruction or duodenal stenosis; biliary tree with jaundice, vascular structures (ie, splenic vein thrombosis), or lymphatic ducts that may result in chylous ascites. Their spontaneous regression is unusual.[14]

Biliary Obstruction

Common bile duct stenosis in patients with chronic pancreatitis occurs in 8% to 46% of patients with chronic pancreatitis and seems to be related to the severity of the disease.[15] No adequate correlation has been noted between the anatomic appearance of obstruction and its functional implications. A clear distinction should be made between acute and persistent hepatic dysfunction. In the former, the pancreas is swollen and edematous, compressing the common bile duct and causing right upper quadrant pain, jaundice, and pruritus. In alcoholic patients this presentation may mimic alcoholic hepatitis. Acute cholangitis is rare, and occurs in less than 5% of cases. Usually the obstruction subsides as inflammation regresses and no specific therapy (drainage) is necessary. In other instances the obstruction is chronic, and results either from fibrosis of the pancreas, including the intrapancreatic segment of the common bile duct, or from pseudocyst compression. Patients may be asymptomatic or have some biochemical abnormalities, such as elevation in the serum concentration of alkaline phosphatase and gamma glutamyl transpeptidase. If they persist and are not treated, biliary cirrhosis may result. This last complication should be suspected when serum alkaline phosphatase remains elevated (more than 2 times normal values) for more than 3 months. These patients should be followed up with serial serum liver tests, cholangiography, and liver biopsies. Portal edema, increased portal fibrosis, and proliferation of interlobular ducts and ductules are commonly found.[16] If progression to cirrhosis is detected, biliary decompression is mandatory. Cholangitis, although an uncommon complication of chronic pancreatitis, may have serious implications, and when diagnosed is an indication for drainage.

Gastrointestinal Hemorrhage

Although serious gastrointestinal bleeding is not common (it occurs in about 10% of cases), it carries a high mortality. Bleeding usually manifests as hematemesis, melena, hematochezia, or a sudden drop in hematocrit, but a chronic blood loss may be observed in some patients. In alcoholic patients it is common to observe gastroduodenal mucosal lesions such as subepithelial hemorrhages, sometimes interpreted as stress ulcers or manifestations of portal hypertension gastropathy. Less frequently, true stress ulcers, gastric and duodenal ulcers, severe esophagitis, or vascular erosions are identified. Two entities deserve special mention: portal hypertension, and aneurysms or pseudoaneurysms. Portal hypertension usually is associated with recurrent episodes of acute pancreatitis with pseudocysts and more rarely with pancreatic tumors. Compression or thrombosis of the splenic, superior mesenteric, and portal veins result in portal hypertension and esophageal, gastric, and sometimes colonic varices. Compression results from edema, expansion, or fibrosis, whereas thrombosis of the splenic vein develops as a consequence of damage to the intima of the vein during inflammatory or neoplastic processes.

Thrombosis of the Splenic Vein

Chronic pancreatitis is the most common cause of isolated thrombosis of the splenic vein. Some of these patients may be asymptomatic, but bleeding occurs in 50% of them. A distinct and diagnostic feature in these patients is the absence of esophageal varices, which occur in less than 10% of all cases. Since it involves the left side of the portal vein system, splenic vein thrombosis is also called "sinistral portal hypertension." Diagnosis of splenic vein thromboses can be suspected in patients with chronic pancreatitis and splenomegaly, upper gastrointestinal hemorrhage, and in those with gastric varices during endoscopy without esophageal varices (Fig. 9.2).

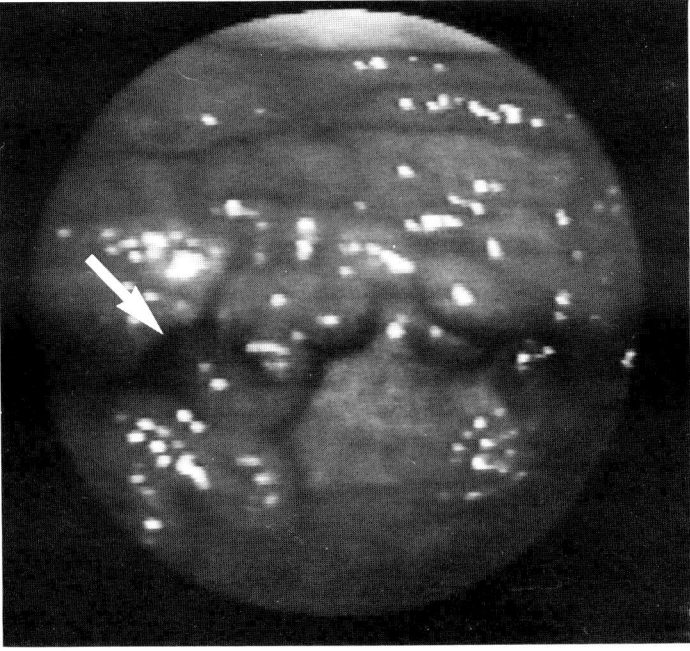

FIGURE 9.2. Large gastric varices in the fundus of the stomach, indicated by blank arrows.

The diagnosis is usually confirmed by Doppler ultrasonography or angiography. In some patients without symptomatic bleeding conservative management is possible because recanalization may take place. In most patients, however, splenectomy is necessary.

Aneurysms and Pseudoaneurysms

Aneurysms may affect the splenic, gastroduodenal, or superior mesenteric arteries, or peripancreatic vessels, and usually result from necrosis and inflammation involving the arterial wall during acute pancreatitis or recurrences of chronic pancreatitis. The aneurysms occur more often in the proximity of a pseudocyst and may hemorrhage into the pseudocyst, resulting in a pseudoaneurysm with increase in the size of the mass. In some instances a bruit may be heard over the mass, and hematocrit and hemoglobin may fall without evidence of external bleeding. In other instances the hemorrhage reaches the duodenum through the pancreatic duct, "hemo succus pancreaticus",[17] and manifests as melena, or less often as hematemesis. In some cases blood may be seen exiting through the papilla during an upper gastrointestinal endoscopy. More often the diagnosis is suspected by ultrasound or CT scan showing changes in size and density of a pseudocyst. Angiography is often diagnostic and also provides the opportunity to embolize the affected vessel in cases with acute bleeding (see Fig. 8.3). If this does not lead to permanent cessation of bleeding, patients should be operated on without delay. The therapy of pseudoaneurysms in chronic pancreatitis is determined by a variety of factors, including the activity of the pancreatic disease, the vessel involved, and the acuteness and severity of bleeding, since in some instances spontaneous resolution has been observed.

Pleural Effusions and Pancreatic Ascites

Although sympathetic pleural effusions may occur in acute pancreatitis, persistent large fluid collections in the pleural space are more characteristic of chronic pancreatitis, usually with a pseudocyst expanding through the diaphragmatic hiatus into the chest. The fluid is characterized by high protein and pancreatic enzyme content (amylase usually greater than 1000 U/dL). Pancreatic ascites results when a pancreatic duct leaks, or a pseudocyst ruptures into the peritoneal cavity.

OTHER CONDITIONS ASSOCIATED WITH CHRONIC PANCREATITIS

Peptic Ulcer Disease

It is generally accepted that patients with chronic pancreatitis may have a slight increased incidence of duodenal ulcers. This is believed to be a result of decreased bicarbonate concentration of the pancreatic juice, which affects its buffer role on duodenal pH.[18] This effect may be aggravated by cigarette smoking, a common habit in chronic alcoholics, since nicotine directly inhibits bicarbonate secretion.

Alcoholic Liver Disease

Chronic alcoholism may affect both the liver and the pancreas. An association between chronic alcoholic pancreatitis and chronic alcoholic liver disease has been recognized. Its prevalence varies according to different series and selection criteria. When changes in liver biopsies are used as criteria, as many as 20% of patients with pancreatitis have liver disease.[19] Autopsy studies of patients dying from alcoholic liver disease reveal that 20% of them are found to have diffuse pancreatic fibrosis or true calcifying pancreatitis.[20]

NATURAL HISTORY

Longitudinal studies of medically and surgically treated chronic pancreatitis patients have provided valuable data for understanding the natural history of this entity.[4] One of the important conclusions is that there are similar results in pain relief when comparison is done between operated and nonoperated patients.[21,22] This may be related more to the duration of the disease leading to progressive pancreatic parenchymal destruction than to results of surgical treatment. The long-term mortality (more than 10 years) is similar in operated compared with nonoperated patients, although in the short term, operated patients have higher mortality due to immediate post operative complications. Finally, about 80% of deaths are caused by extrapancreatic causes, including malignancies, cardiovascular diseases, infections, and nonpancreatic surgery.[23]

FORMS OF CHRONIC PANCREATITIS

Chronic Alcoholic Pancreatitis

There is convincing evidence that alcohol abuse is the major cause of chronic pancreatitis in the Western hemisphere. The pathogenic mechanisms linking excessive alcohol consumption and chronic pancreatitis are not completely understood because most chronic alcoholics (almost 90%) do not develop chronic pancreatitis. Smoking, a common habit among drinkers, has also been thought to contribute. In alcoholics, the first symptoms of pancreatitis appear after 10 or more years of excessive alcohol ingestion, although significant variability has been observed. Women seem to be more susceptible, with shorter periods of alcohol consumption usually seen at the onset of symptoms.[24] Age of onset is between 35 and 40 years, and there is a male predominance ranging from 3:1 to 9:1 in different series. Mean daily alcohol consumption is exponentially related to the risk of developing pancreatitis, with a minimal daily threshold of 40 g/day. Alcohol consumption is usually much greater; daily alcohol intake in patients with chronic alcoholic pancreatitis was 179 g/day compared with 74 g/day in a control population, and their diet contained more protein and fat in one study.[25]

The lesions of chronic alcoholic pancreatitis are distributed unevenly. Some areas are spared entirely, while irregular ductal dilations may affect some segments or the entire length of the main duct. In final stages the gland becomes atrophic and fibrotic. In about one third of the patients the first manifestation of chronic pancreatitis is an acute attack, and recurrence is common during the next 4 to 5 years. The number of acute episodes is roughly related to alcohol consumption; however, no positive correlation has been established between the frequency of recurrent episodes and drinking habits (eg, steady versus "binge" drinkers). During the first 5 years complications such as necrotic pseudocysts and cholestasis frequency occur. Between the fifth and tenth year of disease, the frequency of acute episodes seems to decrease, although the occurrence of pseudocysts (retention pseudocysts) and cholestasis remains high. Beyond the tenth year, the risk of complications that require surgical intervention decreases while acute episodes tend to disappear and pancreatic calcifications, steatorrhea, and diabetes become more prominent. Deterioration of pancreatic function in chronic alcoholic pancreatitis is not always irreversible. In some instances progression is slower and less severe after alcohol abstinence, pancreatic drainage, or both.[4,6,11]

Chronic alcoholic pancreatitis is an entity with high morbidity and relatively low mortality. At 20 years the survival rate is estimated to be about 60%. Most fatal complications occur early in the course of the disease, with late deaths probably resulting from alcoholism and smoking.

SOCIOECONOMIC ASPECTS

Chronic alcoholic pancreatitis is observed more often among the lower socioeconomic groups. It impacts negatively on the capacity of patients to work, and is aggravated by the tendency to develop narcotic dependency. Although Gastard et al observed that the ability to work improves 15 years after the onset of the disease, most patients continue to suffer social discrimination because of the consequences of narcotic addiction and alcoholism rather than pancreatitis.[26]

NUTRITIONAL OR TROPICAL PANCREATITIS

Nutritional pancreatitis has been observed among children and young adults of lower socioeconomic levels in African countries such as Nigeria and in India. The pancreas appears fibrotic with variable degrees of ductal dilation and calculi. Malnutrition has been proposed as a cause, although this is not entirely clear. A positive correlation with consumption of cassava or tapioca (tuber manihot esculenta) has

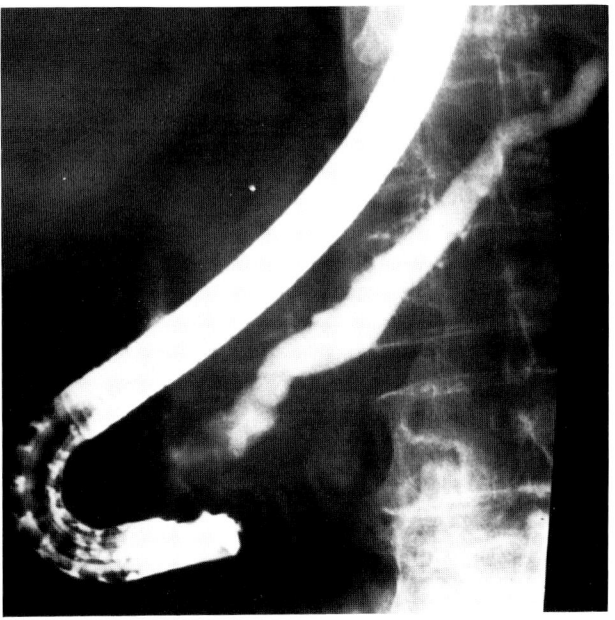

FIGURE 9.3. Endoscopic pancreatogram demonstrates narrowing of the main pancreatic duct (arrow) with uniform dilation distally. The patient had moderate exocrine insufficiency with 12 g/24 h fatty acids in the stools. Endoscopic sphincterotomy was performed and a 12 Fr stent placed. Follow-up revealed disappearance of the steatorrhea.

been observed and it has been proposed that cyanide contained in this root could have a direct toxic effect.[27] Patients have extreme emaciation, parotid gland enlargement, and a distended abdomen. Two thirds of patients complain of abdominal pain, and diabetes becomes predominant in the majority after a few years. Diabetes is usually brittle with episodes of hypoglycemia commonly seen after even small doses of insulin.[28]

OBSTRUCTIVE CHRONIC PANCREATITIS

Obstructive chronic pancreatitis is a distinct form of chronic pancreatitis characterized by dilation of the ductal system proximal to the occlusion of a major duct, with atrophy of the acini and diffuse fibrosis. Pancreatic duct obstruction may result from ampullary fibrosis, papillary inflammation, congenital or acquired strictures of the main duct, or tumors. There is moderate dilation of the main duct, without segmental strictures and dilations. The lesions are microscopically uniform. Calculi are remarkably absent and flow and enzyme secretion markedly decreased. Both morphologic and functional capacities tend to improve when the obstruction is removed (Fig. 9.3).[29]

HEREDITARY CHRONIC PANCREATITIS

A positive family history of chronic pancreatitis in the absence of malnutrition or alcoholism is usually obtained. Patients have recurrent episodes of pain, and pancreatic calcifications are frequently found. Prolonged periods without pain occur, and steatorrhea and diabetes are uncommon.

IDIOPATHIC CHRONIC PANCREATITIS

Idiopathic chronic pancreatitis seems to represent between 10% and 20% of all cases of chronic pancreatitis. It occurs without pain in about 50% of all patients, and has a better survival rate than alcoholic pancreatitis. Two clinical forms are often recognized: juvenile idiopathic pancreatitis, which occurs under the age of 30 and is distinct from cystic fibrosis because of its common association with diabetes and the presence of calcifications; and senile idiopathic pancreatitis, which occurs at a mean age of 65. In senile idiopathic pancreatitis there is a long time lag between the clinical onset, appearance of calcifications, and manifestations of exocrine insufficiency and diabetes (about 15 years, compared with 8 years in alcoholic pancreatitis).

CALCIFIED PANCREATITIS

Detection of pancreatic calcifications has been recognized as a pathognomonic finding of chronic pancreatitis and is considered with steatorrhea and diabetes as representative of advanced stages of the disease. Most of the time the calculi are in the pancreatic ducts and consist of proteinaceous material and calcium carbonate stones (Fig. 9.4). Their incidence varies from 30% to 90%, and although there may be differences in diagnostic criteria and selection of patients, there seem to be true geographical variations, with a higher incidence seen in Europe than in the United States.

Calcified pancreatitis is not a distinct entity and may be found in hypercalcemia, or idiopathic, familial, or hereditary pancreatitis associated with malnutrition, although in Western countries it usually is associated with chronic alcoholism. The lesions are similar regardless of the cause, which suggests a common pathogenic mechanism. Ammann et al proposed three phases in the formation of calcifications in chronic pancreatitis. The initial phase is characterized by gradual increase in calculi formation, with a median time of about 5 years. The second phase is characterized by stabilization in the size of the calcifications. A third, late phase shows decrease and eventual disappearance of the calculi.[23] The mechanism for spontaneous dissolution of calcifications is unknown and it is not known why not all patients with chronic pancreatitis develop calcifications. Lankisch et al observed patients with pancreatic calcifications without pancreatic insufficiency and proposed that the presence of pancreatic calcifications does not necessarily indicate abnormal exocrine function.[29]

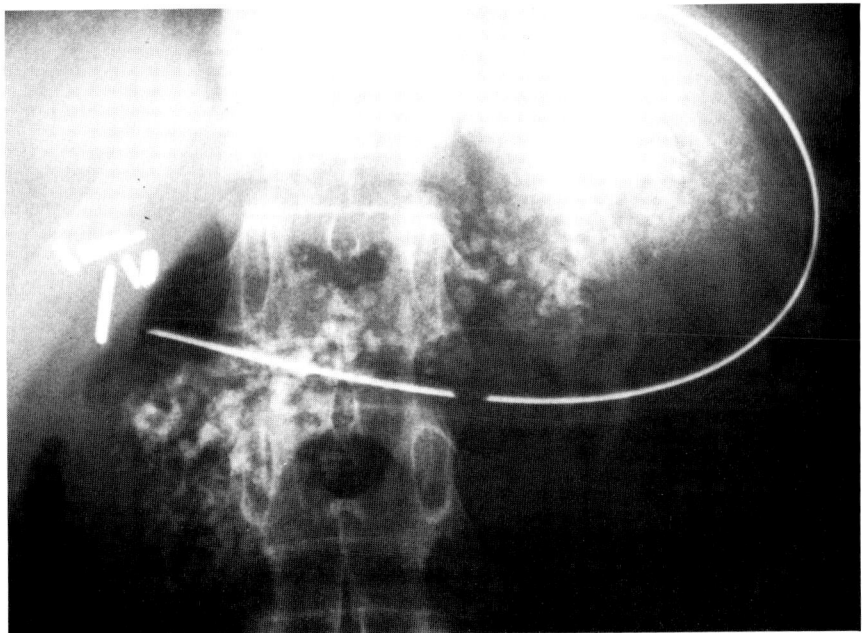

FIGURE 9.4. Abdominal film showing multiple calcifications throughout the head, body, and tail of the pancreas.

References

1. Worning H. Etiologic aspects of chronic pancreatitis. *Int J Pancreatol* 1989;5:1–9.
2. Braganza J, Hunt LP, Warnick F. Relationship between pancreatic exocrine function and ductal morphology in chronic pancreatitis. *Gastroenterology* 1982;82:1341–1347.
3. Kalthoff L, Layer P, Clain JE, et al. The course of alcoholic and non-alcoholic chronic pancreatitis. *Dig Dis Sci* 1984;29:953.
4. Ammann RW, Akovbiantz A, Largiader F, et al. Course and outcome of chronic pancreatitis: longitudinal study of a mixed medical-surgical series of 245 patients. *Gastroenterology* 1984;86:820–828.
5. Hayakawa T, Kondo T, Shibata T, et al. Chronic alcoholism and evolution of pain and prognosis in chronic pancreatitis. *Dig Dis Sci* 1989;34:33–8.
6. Ammann R, Akovbiantz A, Largiader F, et al. Course and outcome of chronic pancreatitis. *Gastroenterology* 1984;86:820–826.
7. Ink O, Labayle D, Buffet C, et al. Pancreatite chronique alcoolique: relations de la douleur avec le sevrage et al chirurgie pancreatique. *Gastroenterol Clin Biol* 1984;8:419–425.
8. Mannel A, Adson MA, McIlrath DC, et al. Surgical management of chronic pancreatitis: long-term results in 141 patients. *Br J Surg* 1988;75:467–472.
9. Ihse I. Pancreatic pain. *Br J. Surg* 1990;77:121–2.
10. Ebbehj N, Borly L, Madsen P, et al. Pancreatic tissue pressure and pain in chronic pancreatitis. *Pancreas* 1986;1:556–8.
11. Bockman D, Buchler M, Malfertheiner P, et al. Analysis of nerves in chronic pancreatitis. *Gastroenterology* 1988;94:1459–1469.

12. Garcia-Puges AM, Navarro S, Ros E, et al. Reversibility of exocrine pancreatic failure in chronic pancreatitis. *Gastroenterology* 1986;91:17–24.
13. Bradley EL, Clement JL, Gonzalez AC. The natural history of pancreatic pseudocysts: a unified concept of management. *Am J Surg* 1979;137:135–140.
14. Bourliever M, Sarles H. Pancreatic cysts and pseudocysts associated with acute and chronic pancreatitis. *Dig Dis Sci* 1989;34:343–348.
15. Petrozza JA, Dutta SK, Latham PS, et al. Prevalence and natural history of distal common bile duct stenosis in alcoholic pancreatitis. *Dig Dis Sci* 1984;29:890–895.
16. Littenberg G, Afrodakis A, Kaplowitz N. Common bile duct stenosis from chronic pancreatitis: a clinical and pathologic spectrum. *Medicine* 1979;58:385–412.
17. Birins BA, Sachatello Cr, Chuang VP, et al. Hemosuccus pancreatitis. *Arch Surg* 1978;113:751–753.
18. Schulze S, Pedersen NT, Jorgensen MJ, et al. Association between duodenal bulb ulceration and reduced exocrine pancreatic function. *Gut* 1983;24:781–783.
19. Renner IG, Savage WT, Stage NH, et al. Pancreatitis associated with alcoholic liver disease: a review of 1022 autopsy cases. *Dig Dis Sci* 1984;29:593–599.
20. Ranson JHC. Acute pancreatitis: pathogenesis, outcome and treatment. *Clin Gastroenterol* 1984;13:843–863.
21. Ink O, Labayle D, Buffet C, et al. Pancreatite chronique alcoolique: relations de la seoleur avec le sevrage et la chiruje pancreatique. *Gastroenterol Clin Biol* 1984;8:419–425.
22. Levy P, Milan C, Pignon JP, et al. Mortality factors associated with chronic pancreatitis. *Gastroenterology* 1989;96:1165–1172.
23. Ammann R, Muench R, Otto R, et al. Evolution and regression of pancreatic calcifications in chronic pancreatitis: a prospective long term study of 107 patients. *Gastroenterology* 1988;95:1018–1128.
24. Mezeye E, Kolman CJ, Diehl AM, et al. Alcohol and dietary intake in the development of chronic pancreatitis and liver disease in alcoholism. *Am J Clin Nutrition* 1988;48:148–151.
25. Sarles H. An international survey on nutrition and pancreatitis. *Digestion* 1973;9:389–403.
26. Gastard J, Joubaud F, Tarbos T, et al. Etiology and course of primary chronic pancreatitis in Western France. *Digestion* 1972;9:416–428.
27. Pitchumoni CS, Jain NK, Lowenfels AB, et al. Chronic cyanide poisoning: unifying concept for alcoholic and tropical pancreatitis. *Pancreas* 1988;3:220–222.
28. Pitchumoni CS. Special problems of tropical pancreatitis. *Clin Gastroenterol* 1984;13:941–959.
29. Lankisch PG, Otto J, Erkelenz I, et al. Pancreatic calcifications: no indicator of severe exocrine insufficiency. *Gastroenterology* 1986;90:617–21.

Chapter 10

Diagnosis of Chronic Pancreatitis

ANDRÉ RIBET
JACQUES MOREAU
JORGE E. VALENZUELA

PANCREATIC FUNCTION TESTS

The pancreas has always been recognized as a difficult organ to access and study. Considerable progress has been achieved in the last 20 years in the assessment of morphologic changes with ultrasonography (US), computerized (CT) scanning, and endoscopic retrograde pancreatography (ERP). Examination of exocrine function remains an important step in the evaluation of patients with suspected chronic pancreatitis. Functional assessment is always referred to as the conventional "gold standard," implying that measurement of bicarbonate and pancreatic enzymes in pancreatic juice constitutes the most accurate method to diagnose pancreatic insufficiency. This is an expensive method that requires a long and unpleasant duodenal intubation. It is performed routinely in highly specialized centers only. This has led to many attempts to replace this technique by noninvasive tests that do not require intubation but provide reliable information on the functional state of the pancreas. The noninvasive tests provide limited information, however, because of considerable functional reserve of the pancreas. Thus significant exocrine insufficiency becomes evident only at late stages. In advanced pancreatitis morphologic changes are evident more often and the diagnosis can be made by noninvasive morphologic methods such as US and CT scan. Conversely, during the early stages of chronic pancreatitis, the morphologic and functional changes may be subtle and undetectable by any of these tests or by even more invasive procedures such as ERP. Assessment of pancreatic secretory changes may lead to the diagnosis. Exploration of pancreatic exocrine function is indicated in the following situations:

1. To diagnose chronic pancreatitis in patients with abdominal pain or steatorrhea.
2. To evaluate progression of exocrine insufficiency or response to therapy.

There are two types of pancreatic function tests.

Tests with Duodenal Intubation

In duodenal intubation the patient fasts overnight and swallows a double lumen tube. The tip is positioned under fluoroscopic guidance in the third portion of the duodenum. Gastric and duodenal secretions are aspirated separately.

Tests with Direct Stimulation of the Pancreas

a) Methods:
Tests that directly stimulate the pancreas measure bicarbonate and pancreatic enzyme concentrations and output in the duodenal content after direct stimulation of the pancreas. Peptides of the cholecystokinin (CCK) family, including natural CCK-33, the synthetic octapeptide (CCK-8) or the decapeptide (Caerulein), and natural or synthetic secretin are used. These peptides stimulate enzyme flow and bicarbonate secretion more selectively.
b) Choice of stimulatory peptides:
Unfortunately there is a lack of uniformity and standardization with these methods, which makes comparisons between the different centers somewhat difficult. Cooperative efforts by the European Pancreatic Club have led to a more standardized procedure.[1-3]

CHOICE OF THE PEPTIDES:

There are two available secretins. One is purified natural porcine secretin (Ferring Laboratories, Inc., Suffern, NY); the other is a synthetic form (Squibb, Princeton, NJ). They have similar potencies and slightly higher bicarbonate response after administration of the synthetic secretin. CCK is available as a partially purified porcine peptide (Kabi Diagnostica, Studsvik, Sweden), as a synthetic CCK-8 (Kinevac, Squibb Diagnostics, New Brunswick, NJ), and caerulein (Farmitalia, Italy). The peptides can be injected sequentially or simultaneously. Giving them together offers the advantage of secretin inhibiting gastric acid secretion, which facilitates collection of pure duodenal content without gastric content contamination. The peptides can also be given as a bolus or by continuous intravenous infusion. When secretin is given as a bolus, a rapid secretory response is observed with peak volume and bicarbonate in the first 10 to 15 minutes. It seems more convenient, however, to infuse the peptides, because maximal doses can be given, which allows better discrimination, and some side effects observed with the bolus administration of secretin (mild transient hypotension) and CCK (abdominal pain, nausea, and vomiting) can be avoided.

Doses recommended in Europe are 0.5 to 1.0 IU/kg/h of secretin and 75 ng/kg/h of caerulein or 40 to 50 ng/kg/h of CCK-8 infused for 60 minutes.[4,5] A small amount of human serum albumin can be added to avoid adherence of the peptides to the plastic syringe or tubing during the infusion.

PANCREATIC JUICE COLLECTION:

Pure pancreatic juice is not indeed collected since duodenal aspiration cannot avoid bile contamination. This is not a major problem except for some bicarbonate contained in the bile. Adequate position of the tube must be assured, however, and continuous and careful aspiration of gastric juice is needed to avoid mixing with duodenal content. The rate of duodenal recovery varies between 65% and 85% and this can be accurately quantitated by perfusing a nonabsorbable marker (eg, polyethylene glycol, isotopes, or dyes) into the duodenum.

Bicarbonate and enzymes (amylase, lipase, trypsin, chymotrypsin) concentrations are determined and output calculated according to the volume of the aspirate.[6]

INTERPRETATION AND DIAGNOSTIC VALUE:

The secretin–CCK test has a sensitivity of 75% to 95% depending on the patient selection criteria. It usually becomes abnormal when there is between 70% and 75% destruction of the parenchyma. Peak bicarbonate concentration and output provide one of the most sensitive indexes. In our experience a peak bicarbonate concentration of more than 90 mEq/L usually rules out the diagnosis of chronic pancreatitis. It is recognized that as many as 10% of patients with proven chronic pancreatitis may have bicarbonate concentration within the normal range, however.[2,7]

Similarly, specificity is determined by the control population selected, the technique used, and the experience of the laboratory. The finding of an abnormal pancreatic secretory response is diagnostic for pancreatic pathology in 80% to 90% of cases. False positive results may be observed among diabetics, (although some of them may have painless chronic pancreatitis), after truncal vagotomy, and in cases with severe malnutrition or malabsorption. The control group must include a wide range of male and female patients of all ages because in women secretion tends to be 20% lower than in men and a decrease in secretion is observed after the age of 70.[2,7] Variations of the secretory tests such as prolonged and repeated stimulation, dose-response infusions, and measurement of enzyme synthesis by administering selenium 75-labeled methionine have only made the tests more cumbersome, more expensive, and have no additional diagnostic value.[8]

Meal-Stimulation Test (Lundh Test)

The Lundh test evaluates pancreatic secretion by measuring tryptic activity in duodenal aspirate after a mixed meal containing 6% fat, 5% protein, and 15% carbohydrates. The sensitivity of the test is less than that of the secretin–CCK test and its specificity is low because factors other than pancreatic secretion such as gastric emptying and duodenogastric reflux affect the results. The best indication for this test is to assess therapeutic results with pancreatic extracts.

Tests with Examination of Pure Pancreatic Juice Obtained by Endoscopic Cannulation

Collection of pure pancreatic juice is ideal but requires endoscopic cannulation of the duct. The procedure is more invasive and expensive, the technique requires considerable experience, and continuous collection of juice is difficult, therefore output cannot be accurately calculated. Cytology of the juice is not a valuable adjunct in the differential diagnosis of pancreatic cancer because of its low sensitivity.

Analysis of Pancreatic Juice

Five to ten minutes after administration of secretin as a bolus or infusion, the flow of pancreatic juice increases rapidly. This juice is characteristically rich in enzyme content and it is believed that this represents enzymes already stored in the ducts, or: a "wash out" effect. Dreiling et al proposed that bicarbonate concentration after secretin is the earliest and more accurate indicator of chronic pancreatitis.[10] More recent experiences have indicated that determination of enzyme output may be of better discriminatory value.[11] This is probably related to the use of CCK. Total protein, amylase, lipase, trypsin, and chymotrypsin are among the enzymes measured most often. In general, measurement of any enzyme is useful because they discriminate between chronic pancreatitis and healthy controls. Determination of total protein, although useful in samples of pure pancreatic juice, is less accurate when duodenal aspirate is obtained, since other nonpancreatic proteins will be included. Abnormal secretion after CCK administration may be observed in chronic alcoholics without pancreatitis, with and without cirrhosis. In alcoholics there is increased protein output, whereas in cirrhotics the flow of juice is augmented.

NONENZYME PROTEINS

LACTOFERRIN: Lactoferrin has a molecular weight of 70,000 d and is normally present in salivary, mammary, bronchial, and pancreatic secretions. Patients with chronic pancreatitis have increased concentrations in pancreatic juice, although its measurement lacks the specificity and sensitivity to recommend its determination as a routine diagnostic test.[12]

PANCREATIC STONE PROTEIN

Pancreatic stone protein is decreased in the pancreatic juice of patients with chronic pancreatitis and may play a pathogenic role in calculi formation. The values often overlap those found in nonpancreatitis subjects, however, therefore it has limited diagnostic usefulness.

TUMOR MARKERS: Several tumor markers have been searched for in both duodenal aspirate and pure pancreatic juice in an attempt to identify a diagnostic test for early pancreatic cancer. Carcinoembryogenic antigen (CEA) and CA 19-9 are among the most widely tested. Contrary to study of CA 19-9 in serum, study of tumor markers in pancreatic juice has been disappointing.[13]

Tubeless (Noninvasive) Tests

Noninvasive tests can be grouped according to the functional derangement they detect. In some a synthetic substrate relatively specific for a pancreatic hydrolase is given orally and the test molecule, which can only be absorbed after hydrolysis, is measured in the blood or urine. The para-amino benzoic (PABA) test, pancreolauryl test, and the modified Schilling test are among these types of tests. A variant of these tests is to label the substrate so that after hydrolysis a labeled diffusible gas such as $[^{14}C]$-carbon dioxide can be measured in the expired breath. The triolein test is an example of such a test.

A second category of nonintrusive tests evaluates the amount of a nutrient reaching the colon after incomplete digestion. In some tests the nutrients are directly measured in the stools (eg, fatty acids or nitrogen) to indicate the presence of steatorrhea or creatorrhea, respectively. In other tests the undigested substrate reaches the colon, where it undergoes bacterial hydrolysis to generate H_2, which is then measured in the breath. A third group of tests assesses pancreatic enzymes in the urine or stools, and in a fourth group of tests, pancreatic peptides are measured in the blood to reflect the degree of endocrine cell parenchymal destruction as an index of chronic pancreatitis.

NBT-PABA (Bentiromide) Test

N-benzoyl-1-tyrosyl-para-aminobenzoic acid (NBT-PABA) is a synthetic tripeptide that yields free PABA after hydrolysis by chymotrypsin. The PABA is absorbed by the intestinal mucosa, conjugated in the liver, and excreted in the urine. The serum concentration of PABA and the total amount eliminated in the urine is compared with the amount ingested and reflects exocrine pancreatic function. Healthy subjects eliminate more than 50% of PABA in the urine.[14]

METHOD:

NBT-PABA (Hoffman-La Roche, Grenzach, Germany) is given with a standardized meal. The patient also drinks about 500 mL of water or tea. Urine recovery of PABA is determined over 6 hours. Pancreatic extracts and drugs that might interfere with PABA elimination are withheld for the 5 days preceding the test. The test has a sensitivity of about 85% and specificity of about 75% depending on the selection criteria. When the NBT-PABA test is done in patients with chronic pancreatitis who have diarrhea, steatorrhea, or weight loss the test will be abnormal in more than 90% of them. Conversely, if these symptoms are absent, the test may be normal in most patients. Intestinal, hepatic, and renal diseases can affect the results. NTB-PABA proteolysis can be carried by intestinal bacteria and cause false negative results after gastric surgery or in cases of bacterial overgrowth. About 50% of diabetic patients exhibit abnormal results.

Some modifications have been introduced to improve the specificity of the test, such as measurement of PABA blood levels, repeating the test 48 hours later, giving PABA, or administering NBT-PABA together with labeled [^{14}C] PABA.[15,16] There seems to be little gain by these modifications.

Pancreolauryl Test

In the pancreolauryl test (PTL) the substrate fluorescein dilaurate (Pancreolauryl, Temmler, Marburg, Germany) is hydrolyzed by a pancreatic esterase to yield fluorescein, which is readily absorbed from the intestine, conjugated in the liver, and excreted in the urine. Diuresis is stimulated by giving water or tea for the next 3 to 5 hours. Fluorescein can be measured in the serum or in the urine, which is collected for 10 hours. The test is repeated 48 hours later with free fluorescein to correct for intestinal absorption, liver failure, and urinary function. Fluorescein in the serum or urine during the test day (T) and the control day (C) is expressed as the ratio T:C. A ratio higher than 30% is considered normal and one lower than 20% is indicative of pancreatic dysfunction. Ratios between 20% and 30% are not diagnostic and the test must be repeated. If repeated values fall in the same range, the test is considered abnormal.[16,17] Measurement of fluorescein in the serum shortens the test considerably. The best discriminatory serum value is observed at 210 minutes with a cut-off serum fluorescein concentration of 1.5 μg/mL.

Compared with the secretin–CCK test, the PLT test sensitivity is about 80% for severe chronic pancreatitis and 40% for moderate cases. The PLT test has a sensitivity similar to that of the bentiromide test, although the specificity appears to be somewhat lower.

Dual-Labeled Schilling Test

Vitamin B12 binds to protein R in saliva and gastric juice and binds to intrinsic factor only after proteases partially degrade protein R. In cases of severe pancreatitis, vitamin B12 remains bound to protein R, cannot bind completely to intrinsic factor, and is not absorbed in the ileum. Patients may have an abnormal Schilling test. This is not specific for pancreatic insufficiency. In a modified version, the dual-labeled Schilling test, [^{57}Co]cobalamin bound to intrinsic factor and [^{58}Co]cobalamin bound to protein R are given together and elimination of both is measured in the urine during 24 hours. In healthy subjects both forms are absorbed, while in patients with pancreatic insufficiency the ratio of ^{58}Co to ^{57}Co is low. In patients with intestinal causes of malabsorption, the absorption of both isotopes is affected and the ratio is normal. This test appears to have good sensitivity and correlates well with results obtained with the secretin–CCK test.[18]

Labeled-Lipid Tests

TRIOLEIN BREATH TEST:

The triolein breath test is a two-stage test based on elimination of [^{14}C] carbon dioxide in the breath after ingestion of labeled triolein and a standard breakfast. Triolein that is not hydrolyzed by pancreatic lipase reaches the lower intestine and bacteria digest the lipids, liberating [^{14}C] carbon dioxide. This test is considered a substitute for fecal fat determination. False positive results can be seen in cases of intestinal causes of malabsorption, hepatic failure, and diabetes mellitus. The triolein breath test has low sensitivity and is usually normal in cases with chronic pancreatitis without steatorrhea, but has the disadvantage of radiation exposure, which limits its use in children.

TRIGLYCERIDES AND LABELED FREE FATTY ACIDS:

The triglycerides test examines intraduodenal lipolytic activity by administering a double-labeled [^{14}C]triolein and [^{3}H]oleate meal. Curves of isotopes concentration in the blood are determined for 2 hours. Variants of these tests have been introduced. In one test ^{14}C-labeled triglyceride is used as a substrate, and a more recent version uses a ^{13}C-labeled medium-chain fatty acid in the 2 position and a long-chain fatty acid labeled in the 1 and 3 positions. The rationale behind this test is that the two stearyl groups have to be hydrolyzed by lipase before [^{13}C]octanoyl monoglyceride or [^{13}C]octanoate can be absorbed and metabolized to [^{13}C] carbon dioxide.[19] A third test uses cholesteryloctanoate to analyze expired [^{14}C] carbon dioxide.[20-22] Initial evaluation of these tests suggests that they are good, noninvasive, and provide data comparable with that obtained by direct lipase determination in the intestinal content. Abnormal test results may occur in patients who have metabolic and hepatic diseases and in some diabetics who have delayed gastric emptying.

Measurement of Fat in the Stools

Increased fat in the stools can be determined qualitatively by Sudan stain in a stool sample obtained by digital examination of the rectum without lubrication. It has low sensitivity and specificity. A quantitative determination described by Van de Kamer et al almost 40 years ago has become universally accepted as the standard for steatorrhea.[21] Subjects ingest a high lipid diet (70 to 100 g/day for 3 to 6 days). Steatorrhea is defined as elimination of 7 g or more per 24 hours.[23] This test is not specific for pancreatic insufficiency and therefore has low specificity in the diagnosis of chronic pancreatitis. It has been proposed, however, that high fecal fat excretion is observed more frequently in chronic pancreatitis compared with patients who have steatorrhea after gastric resection or small bowel disease.[24]

Hydrogen Breath Test

The hydrogen breath test is simple and consists of measurement of hydrogen in the breath after ingestion of a rice-flour meal. Breath hydrogen is significantly higher in patients with pancreatic insufficiency, and if normalized by addition of pancreatic extracts, is accurate in diagnosing advanced pancreatic insufficiency. Its yield in the diagnosis of moderate pancreatitis is limited.[24]

Determination of Pancreatic Enzymes

SERUM TRYPSINOGEN:

Pancreatic enzymes usually are determined in the serum or urine to diagnose acute pancreatitis, but determination of serum trypsinogen by radioimmunoassay (Trypsik, CIS-kit, Sorin Biomedica, Saluggia, Vercelli, Italy) can be helpful in the diagnosis of chronic pancreatitis. Although there is overlapping of the values obtained in patients with chronic pancreatitis compared with controls, about 50% of patients with chronic pancreatitis have values below the lower limit of normal (10.3 ng/mL). The test has a low sensitivity but adequate specificity, and a finding of low levels of serum trypsinogen strongly suggests chronic pancreatitis.[25] A modification of this test is administration of bombesin followed by serum and urine determinations of trypsinogen.[26]

FECAL CHYMOTRYPSINOGEN:

Measurement of chymotrypsinogen in the stools has been done for over 20 years. It shows adequate correlation with the protease concentration in duodenal aspirate and fat in the stools. The test has a sensitivity of about 66% for moderate secretory insufficiency and 91% for advanced severe pancreatitis. Specificity varies between 73% and 89%.[26]

Plasma Profile of Pancreatic Hormones

Plasma profile of pancreatic peptides may be affected by the parenchymal destruction that occurs in chronic pancreatitis. Low levels of serum insulin can be detected, and this may affect glycoregulation. In addition serum levels of peptides such as pancreatic polypeptide (PP), produced almost exclusively by endocrine pancreatic cells, may be affected. Low basal levels of serum PP have been observed in patients with chronic pancreatitis, although this finding has a low sensitivity, since almost 35% of healthy subjects may have low serum PP. Conversely, basal plasma levels higher than 125 pM are unlikely in patients with advanced chronic pancreatitis. Because serum levels of PP increase after a meal or after administration of secretin or CCK the sensitivity of the test may be enhanced. No strict correlation has been found between the level of exocrine insufficiency and the postprandial serum PP increment, however. It has been noted that patients with moderate pancreatitis may have a paradoxically higher increment after a meal.[27] This test appears to have limited value and may be reliable only in advanced cases of pancreatitis.

ROLE OF PANCREATIC FUNCTION TESTS

In the Diagnosis of Chronic Pancreatitis

The selection of a function test must be based on clinical grounds to diagnose chronic pancreatitis. For instance, in patients with steatorrhea examination of the exocrine pancreatic function with tubeless tests seems appropriate. Direct examination of the secretory capacity by duodenal intubation and secretin–CCK administration should be reserved for cases with unclear results after noninvasive testing or in moderate cases without steatorrhea. About 10% of patients with chronic pancreatitis may have secretory abnormalities, whereas all morphologic studies including ERP may be normal. Conversely, up to 10% of patients with chronic pancreatitis, including pancreatic calcifications, may have normal secretin–CCK tests.

There are patients with mild chronic pancreatitis without any detectable abnormalities on functional or morphologic studies. In these patients, noninvasive tests are not helpful and a definitive diagnosis can only be made as the disease progresses and more definitive abnormalities occur.

CASE PRESENTATION

A 26-year-old woman without a history of alcohol consumption who had insulin-dependent diabetes was referred for investigation for weight loss, diarrhea, and possible steatorrhea. There was negative family history of pancreatitis or diabetes. She denied abdominal pain, and there was no evidence of peripheral neuropathy or symptoms of gastroparesis. Gallbladder ultrasound was reported as normal. There were no calcifications in the area of the pancreas on the abdominal series. Endoscopic retrograde pancreatography was done and reported as normal. Fatty acids in the stools were increased to 20 g/24 hours and a breath test ruled out the possibility of intestinal bacterial overgrowth.

A secretin–CCK test was performed. After administration of secretin (1 U/kg) the volume was 1.2 mL/kg (normal >1.0 mL/kg); peak bicarbonate was 65 mEq/L (normal >90 mEq/L). After CCK-8 (75 ng/kg) the amylase output was 4800 U/30 minutes (normal >25,000 U/30 minutes).

These results are compatible with advanced pancreatic insufficiency. The patient was placed on enzyme replacement therapy. She gained weight and the insulin therapy was adjusted.

Differential Diagnosis Between Chronic Pancreatitis and Pancreatic Cancer

Functional and pancreatic secretory tests are of limited value in the differential diagnosis between chronic pancreatitis and pancreatic cancer. Clinical information and morphologic examination using US, CT scan, and ERCP appear to provide more valuable information. Examination of the cytology obtained during duodenal aspiration or direct pancreatic duct cannulation adds little to the sensitivity, which is about 50%, although the specificity is about 90%.

Follow-up and Management of Patients with Chronic Pancreatitis

Tubeless tests more accurately assess the pharmacologic response to replacement therapy with pancreatic extracts.

RELATIONSHIP BETWEEN PANCREATIC SECRETORY STUDIES AND IMAGING IN CHRONIC PANCREATITIS

Earlier studies comparing ERCP and secretin–CCK tests indicated similar results, although no strict correlation on the analysis of individual cases could be made.[28]

Subsequently it became more evident that the discrepancy is higher in earlier stages of chronic pancreatitis. In general, as pancreatic insufficiency becomes more accentuated, pancreatic duct abnormalities also become more evident. For instance, most patients with severe ductal abnormalities shown by ERCP have severe secretory insufficiency shown by secretin–CCK testing, whereas in less advanced cases the correlation is lower. Special consideration should be given to patients with chronic obstructive pancreatitis. In these patients differentiation based on morphologic findings between chronic pancreatitis and pancreatic cancer may be particularly difficult. In pancreatic cancer cases, after secretin–CCK testing the volume may be low with normal enzyme concentration because some normal functional parenchyma is present proximal to the tumor. If serum enzymes are monitored, elevated levels may be observed. In contrast, in patients with chronic pancreatitis the low volume may be associated with low enzyme concentration in duodenal juice and absence of enzyme increment in the serum may be detected.

A sequence of imaging studies and tests to identify chronic pancreatitis is presented in the following algorithm. This sequence should diagnose more than 95% of patients with chronic pancreatitis.

Algorithm for Diagnosis of Chronic Pancreatitis

Step 1: Abdominal pain, history of alcoholism; weight loss, steatorrhea, and/or diabetes (one or all are present)

Step 2: Plain abdominal film or US: Pancreatic calcifications

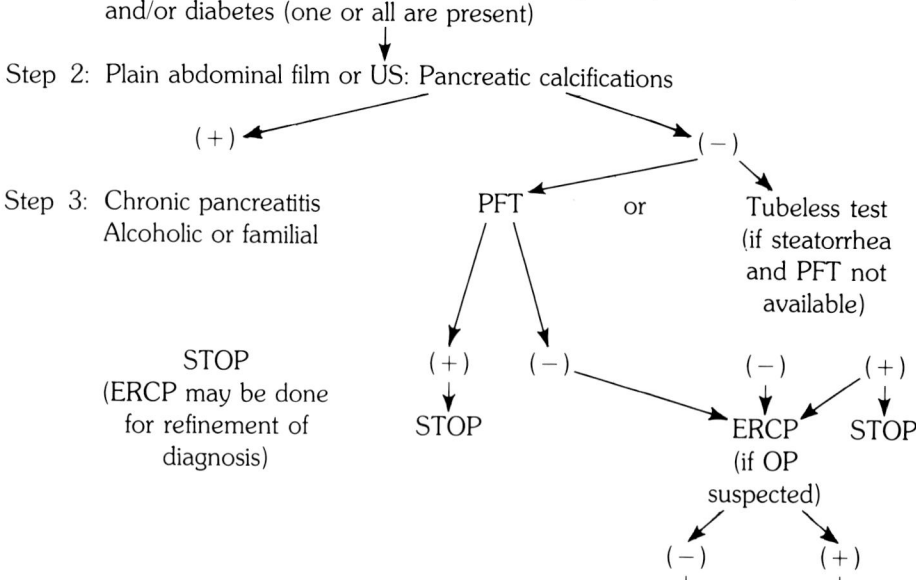

Step 4: If both PFT and ERP are negative follow up and reevaluate

PFT, pancreatic function test with duodenal intubation; ERCP, endoscopic retrograde cholangio pancreatography; OP, obstructive pancreatitis.

References

1. Boyd EJS, Wormsley KG. Part I. Secretagogues used in tests of pancreatic secretion. *Int J Pancreatol* 1987;2:137–148.
2. Boyd EJS, Wormsley KG. Part II. Tests of pancreatic secretion. *Int J Pancreatol* 1987; 2:211–221.
3. Niederau C, Grendell J. Diagnosis of chronic pancreatitis. *Gastroenterology* 1985; 88:1973–1995.
4. Ribet A, Tournut R, Duffaut M, et al. Use of cerulein with subnormal doses as a test of pancreatic function in man. *Gut* 1976;17:431–434.
5. Gullo L. Direct pancreatic function test (duodenal intubation) in the diagnosis of chronic pancreatitis. *Gastroenterology* 1986;90:799–801.
6. Go VLM, DiMagno EP. Assessment of exocrine pancreatic function by duodenal intubation. *Clin Gastroenterol* 1984;13:701–715.
7. Vellas B, Balas D, Moreau J, et al. Exocrine pancreatic secretion in the elderly. *Int J Pancreatol* 1988;3:497–502.
8. Braganza JM, Critchley M, Howat HT, et al. An evaluation of 75 selenomethionine scanning as a test of pancreatic function: a comparison with the secretin-pancreozymin test. *Gut* 1973;14:383–389.
9. Escourrou J, Frexinos J, Ribet A. Biochemical studies of pancreatic juice collected by duodenal aspiration and endoscopic cannulation of the main pancreatic duct. *Dig Dis Sci* 1978;23:173–177.
10. Dreiling DA, Greenstein AJ, Boraldo O. Comparison of standard and augmented secretin tests responses in patient with and without pancreatic disease. *Am J Gastroenterol* 1974; 61:433–443.
11. Multingner L, Figarella C, Sarles H. Diagnosis of chronic pancreatitis by measurement of lactoferrin in duodenal juice. *Gut* 1981;22:350–354.
12. Multigner L, Sarles H, Lombardo D, et al. Pancreatic stone protein: implication in stone formation during the course of chronic calcifying pancreatitis. *Gastroenterology* 1985; 89:387–391.
13. Schmiegel WH, Eberl W, Kreiker C, et al. Multiparametric tumor marker (CA 19-9, CEA, AFP, POA) analyses of pancreatic juices and sera in pancreatic disease. *Hepatogastroenterology* 1985;32:141–145.
14. Lang C, Gyr K, Tonko I, et al. Value of serum PABA as a pancreatic function test. *Gut* 1984;25:508–512.
15. Tanner AR, Robinson DP. Pancreatic function testing: serum PABA measurement is a reliable and accurate measurement of exocrine function. *Gut* 1988;29:1736–1740.
16. Lankisch PG, Schreiber A, Otto J. Pancreolauryl test: evaluation of a tubeless test in comparison with other indirect and direct tests for exocrine pancreatic function. *Dig Dis Sci* 1983;28:490–493.
17. Lankisch PG, Brauneis J. Otto J, et al. Pancreolauryl and NBT-PABA Tests: are serum tests more practicable alternatives to urine tests in the diagnosis of exocrine pancreatic insufficiency? *Gastroenterology* 1986;90:350–354.
18. Brugge WR, Goldberg HJ, Burke CA, et al. Use of pancreatic Schilling test to determine efficiency of pancreatic enzyme delivery in pancreatic insufficiency. *Dig Dis Sci* 1988; 33:1226–1232.
19. Ghoos YF, Vantrappen GR, Rutgeor PJ, et al. A mixed highly triglyceride breath test for fat digestive activity. *Digestion* 1981;22:239–247.

20. Vantrappen GR, Rutgeorts PJ, Ghoos YT, et al. Mixed triglyceride breath test: a noninvasive test of pancreatic lipase activity in the duodenum. *Gastroenterology* 1989;98:1126–1134.
21. Van de Kamer JH, Huinink HB, Weyers HA. Rapid method for the determination of fat in feces. *J Biol Chem* 1949;177:347–355.
22. Bo-Linn G, Fordtran J. Fecal fat concentration in patients with steatorrhea. *Gastroenterology* 1984;87:319–322.
23. Maelue RD, Levine AS, Levitt MD. Malabsorption of starch in pancreatic insufficiency. *Gastroenterology* 1981;80:1220.
24. Andriulli A, Masoero G, Fico O, et al. Evocative test of serum pancreatic enzymes to bombesin in chronic pancreatitis. *Am J Gastroenterol* 1986;81:562–565.
25. Audriulli A, Masoero G, Felder M, et al. Circulating trypsin-like immunoreactivity in chronic pancreatitis. *Dig Dis Sci* 1981;26:532–537.
26. Ammann RW, Akovbiants A, Hacki W, et al. Diagnostic value for the fecal chymotrypsin test in pancreatic insufficiency, particularly chronic pancreatitis: correlation with the Pancreozymin-Secretin test, fecal fat excretion and final clinical diagnosis. *Digestion* 1981;21:21–29.
27. Owyang C, Scarpello JH, Vinik AI. Correlation between pancreatic enzyme secretion and plasma concentration of human pancreatic polypeptide in health and chronic pancreatitis. *Gastroenterology* 1982;83:55–62.
28. Braganza JM, Hunt LP, Warwick F. Relationship between pancreatic exocrine function and ductal morphology in chronic pancreatitis. *Gastroenterology* 1982;82:1341–1347.

Chapter 11

Radiology in Chronic Pancreatitis

PHILIP W. RALLS
HARTLEY COHEN

Plain radiographs have real but limited use in the diagnosis and management of patients with chronic pancreatitis. In patients with uncomplicated chronic pancreatitis, the only finding may be pancreatic calcifications on abdominal plain film, which is highly suggestive of alcoholic pancreatitis. Calcifications related to chronic pancreatitis are seen on plain films in a minority of patients. Computed tomography (CT) is more sensitive in the detection of these calcifications (Fig. 11.1). Chest radiographs are usually normal. Abnormalities on upper gastrointestinal series related to enlargement or fibrosis of the pancreas may be seen, manifested as a duodenal luminal or mucosal mass or irregularity.

Real-time sonography may be useful in patients with chronic pancreatitis. It can detect pancreatic and biliary ductal dilation and may demonstrate intrapancreatic calcifications (Fig. 11.2). Sonography is less sensitive than CT or plain radiography in the detection of calcifications related to chronic pancreatitis. In the absence of calcifications (about 50% of cases), the sonographic diagnosis of chronic pancreatitis may be difficult. Pancreatic ductal dilation, especially when multiple ducts are involved, and focal pancreatic atrophy may suggest the diagnosis. Masses related to chronic pancreatitis are common and may be difficult to differentiate from pancreatic carcinoma, especially if calcifications are absent. Other signs that may prove useful in differentiating masses related to chronic pancreatitis from pancreatic carcinoma include pancreatic ductal dilation distal to the mass or multiple dilated small ducts within the mass.

CT is generally superior to sonography in its ability to image the pancreas since it is not limited by gas-filled bowel loops, which may partially or completely obscure the pancreas. Approximately 90% of patients with chronic pancreatitis have abnormalities on CT. The most frequent of these include dilation of the pancreatic duct (approximately 66%), pancreatic parenchymal and ductal calcification (approximately 50%), pancreatic atrophy (approximately 50%), focal pancreatic enlargement (30%), and bile duct dilation (30%). Another fairly common finding is pancreatic pseudocyst, which may be present in as many as 20% of patients who have no evidence of concomitant acute pancreatitis.

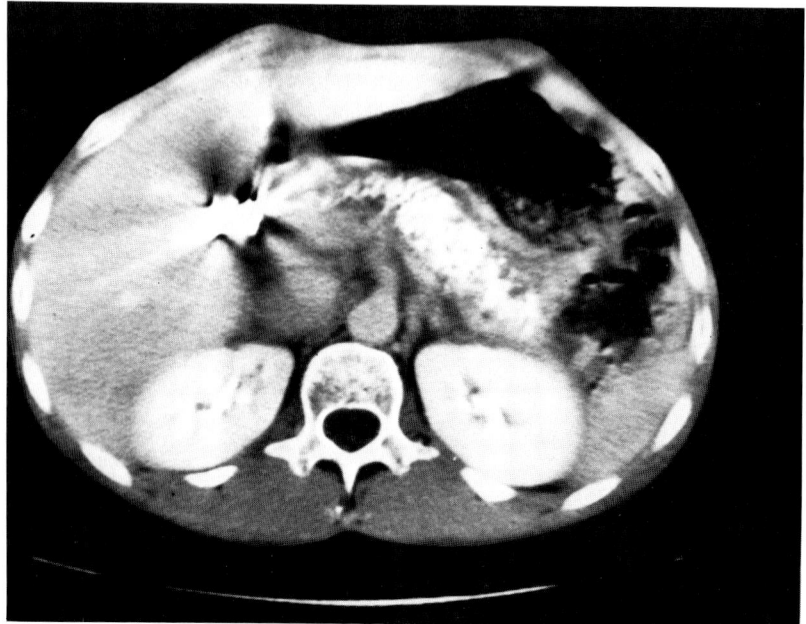

FIGURE 11.1. CT of the abdomen shows multiple calcifications of the pancreas.

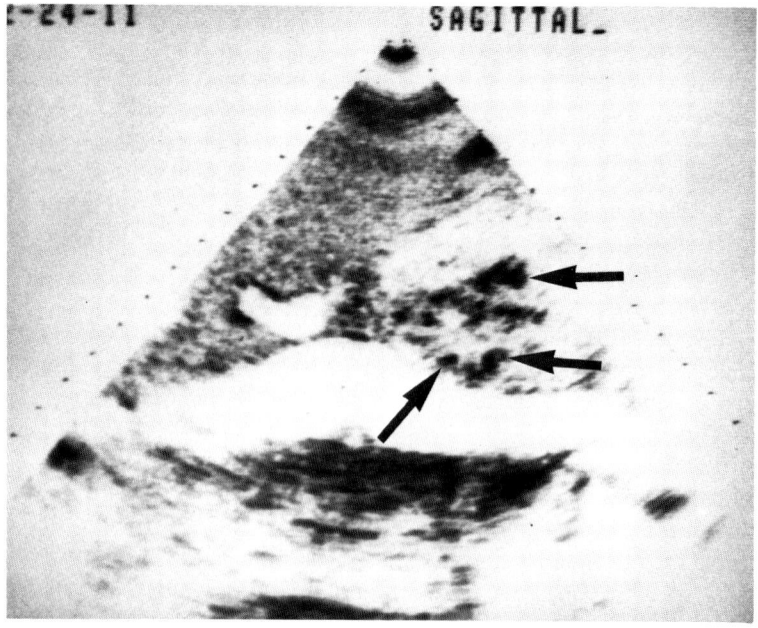

FIGURE 11.2. Pancreatic sonogram shows an enlarged pancreatic head indenting the inferior vena cava. Arrows indicate some of the pancreatic calcifications in a patient with chronic pancreatitis.

CT is of limited use as a diagnostic technique in patients with exocrine insufficiency. Atrophy, as shown by CT, does not correlate well with exocrine insufficiency. In the series by Luetmer et al, only 41% of patients with exocrine insufficiency had severe atrophy, whereas 32% of patients had no atrophy at all.[1] This is not totally surprising since patients with exocrine insufficiency may have normal pancreatic ducts at endoscopic retrograde cholangiopancreatography (ERCP). Four of 22 patients with exocrine insufficiency had completely normal CT, without evidence of calcification atrophy or ductal dilation.

Focal masses are common in patients with chronic pancreatitis, probably much more so than diffuse pancreatic enlargement. If calcifications are present within the mass or if there are dilated ducts in the mass or distal to it, the mass can be safely attributed to chronic pancreatitis. Although it has been reported, chronic calcific pancreatitis is rarely associated with pancreatic carcinoma. In the series by Luetmer, approximately one third of masses associated with chronic pancreatitis could not be differentiated from pancreatic carcinoma.[1] The use of percutaneous biopsy in this setting is somewhat limited as well, since it is really helpful only when biopsy is positive.

ERCP IN CHRONIC PANCREATITIS

ERCP can demonstrate morphologic features of the main pancreatic duct and the major side branches. These features can be categorized either as normal, or as mildly, moderately, or severely abnormal changes characteristic of chronic pancreatitis (Fig. 11.3).

ERCP in patients with chronic pancreatitis, as in those with pancreatic carcinoma, is probably the most sensitive and specific diagnostic test. This conclusion is based on studies comparing the accuracy of different imaging modalities with each other and with results of pancreatic function testing. Unfortunately, the available literature comparing these diagnostic modalities with one another is difficult to interpret due to the heterogeneity of patients studied and because only some of the modalities were evaluated in the different reports. Thus, comparisons between these studies are hazardous. Moreover, technologic improvements in ultrasonographic and CT scanning equipment may render earlier studies irrelevant. The evidence suggesting that ERCP is the most accurate test for the diagnosis of chronic pancreatitis therefore is not clear cut, but is selectively summarized as follows. In a carefully performed study, pancreatic function tests were performed in a group of patients to measure the volume and secretion of bicarbonate, lipase, and chymotrypsin output after secretin and cholecystokinin stimulation, and these results were compared with pancreatic ultrasonographic findings. Only three quarters of the patients with abnormal functional tests were found to have morphologic alterations detected ultrasonographically.[2] Thus, pancreatic function tests were found to be more accurate than ultrasonography for the diagnosis of chronic pancreatitis. Pancreatic function tests also were found to be more accurate than ERCP in an earlier study by the same group.[3] In other studies, however, ERCP was found to be equal to or more sensitive than pancreatic function tests in detecting chronic pancreatitis.[4,5] In other studies, CT scanning is either more or less sensitive

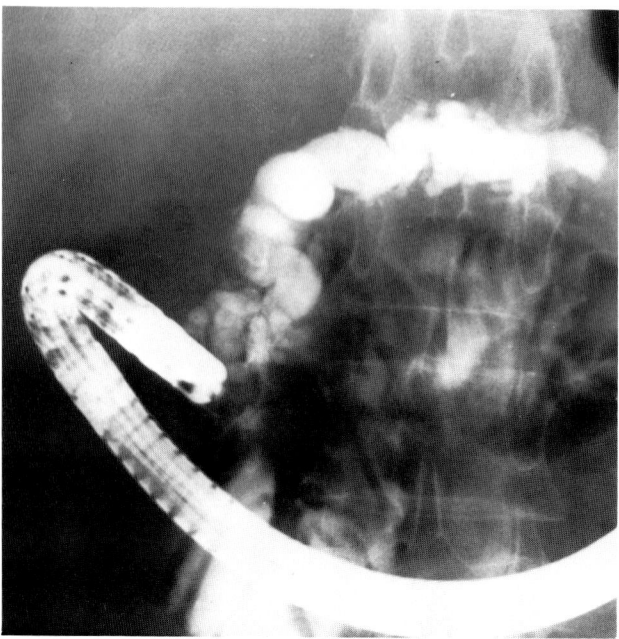

FIGURE 11.3. Pancreatogram shows severe changes with dilated main pancreatic duct and lateral side branches with irregularities.

than ERCP in documenting chronic pancreatitis. The differences in sensitivity among CT studies, ultrasonographic evaluations, pancreatic function tests, and ERCP are very small, however.

How should the clinician evaluate a patient with suspected chronic pancreatitis? A reasonable algorithm for the diagnosis of chronic pancreatitis is to begin with an abdominal film or ultrasonography (see algorithm in chapter 10), since this is noninvasive and the latter test does not have the disadvantage of ionizing radiation. If this study is indeterminant, a CT scan can be performed. If this also results in indeterminant findings, it is reasonable to perform an ERCP. Pancreatic function tests are available in few centers and therefore are not routinely recommended. ERCP, however, may be normal in as many as 20% of patients who have mildly abnormal function tests. Thus, there is no single "gold standard" for the diagnosis of chronic pancreatitis. For practical purposes, however, the previously outlined algorithm for the diagnosis of chronic pancreatitis should allow a diagnosis to be made in more than 90% of patients.

In addition to its value in diagnosis, ERCP also can be used for therapeutic purposes in chronic pancreatitis. This is presently an evolving area and only a few patients have been treated. Nonetheless, enthusiasts claim amelioration of pain using the techniques of endoscopic pancreatic sphincterotomy, sometimes associated with the removal of pancreatic duct stones, and sometimes with the placement of a stent within the pancreatic duct. These studies have been uncontrolled, however, and some concern has been voiced regarding the possibility of inducing morphologic pancreatic duct changes by the placement of a pancreatic stent. These latter changes probably are transient, and most likely related to stent clogging or trauma at the time of stent removal. Ideally, placement of pancreatic stents or performance of pancreatic sphincterotomies should be done in the setting of a controlled trial to further evaluate the efficacy of these procedures.

There is limited experience in treating pancreatic pseudocysts with an endoscopic technique (see pages 78–80). In cases where there is close apposition between the cyst and the intestinal wall, a puncture (using a diathermic needle) is made, either between the gastric or duodenal lumen and the cyst. The opening is enlarged to about 1 cm and a nasocystic drain or a stent may be placed across the opening to ensure continued communication between the cyst and the intestinal lumen. In the duodenum, a side-viewing endoscope is used most frequently, but for a cyst gastrostomy a forward-viewing endoscope also may be used. Endoscopic ultrasonography may be employed initially to ascertain the proximity of the cyst to the duodenal or gastric wall. Most of the experience with this technique has been reported from European centers, and most of them claim excellent results (resolution of the cysts and pain relief). There is limited experience in the United States. As is usual with most novel approaches, early reports document good results. More experience is necessary before this technique can be recommended. Randomized comparative studies of observation (conservative management), endoscopic drainage, and percutaneous drainage would be helpful in delineating the role of these modalities, as compared to standard surgical treatment.

References

1. Luetmer PH, Stephens DH, Ward EM. Chronic pancreatitis: reassessment with current CT. *Radiology* 1989;171:353–357.
2. Bolondi L, Priori P, Gullo L, et al. Relationship between morphological changes detected by ultrasonography and pancreatic exocrine function in chronic pancreatitis. *Pancreas* 1987; 2:222–229.
3. Caletti G, Brocchi E, Agostini D, et al. Sensitivity of endoscopic retrograde pancreatology in chronic pancreatitis. *Br J Surg* 1982;69:507–509.
4. Malfertheiner P, Buchler M, Stanescu A, et al. Exocrine pancreatic function in correlation to ductal and parenchymal morphology in chronic pancreatitis. *Hepatogastroenterology* 1986;33:110–114.
5. Mee AS, Girwood AH, Walker E, et al. Comparison of the oral (PABA) pancreatic function test, the secretin-pancreozymin test and endoscopic retrograde pancreatography in chronic alcohol induced pancreatitis. *Gut* 1985;26:1257–1262.

Chapter 12

Treatment of Chronic Pancreatitis

ANDRÉ RIBET
JACQUES MOREAU
JORGE E. VALENZUELA
HOWARD A. REBER
NARIMAN D. KARANJIA

The goals of treatment for chronic pancreatitis are pain relief; correction of malabsorption and its consequences, steatorrhea and weight loss; and maintenance of blood sugar control.

ABDOMINAL PAIN

The mechanism of pain in chronic pancreatitis is not known. Some of the causes that need to be evaluated in each patient are:

Continued Alcohol Ingestion

It is generally recognized that painful episodes occur closely related to alcohol ingestion and it is assumed that this is due to the stimulatory effect of alcohol on pancreatic secretion. The available information is somewhat conflicting, however. For instance, the direct effect of alcohol on pancreatic secretion is complex. First, alcohol is a mild stimulant of acid secretion and indirectly may stimulate the pancreas by secretin release. Second, when alcohol is given intragastrically into the intestine or intravenously, inhibition of pancreatic enzyme secretion is observed in healthy subjects. Third, this inhibitory effect is not observed in chronic alcoholics. Fourth, there is evidence that some alcoholic beverages such as beer and wine have a stimulatory effect presumedly caused by the nonalcoholic components of these beverages.[1] Regardless of the net effect of alcohol or alcoholic beverages on the pancreas, clinical observations seem to suggest that episodes of pain are often observed shortly after alcohol ingestion. Certainly the influence of heavy meals eaten while drinking cannot be ignored. Some clinical series report disappearance of pain in patients who become abstinent.[2] Some surgical series suggest that abstinence enhances pain relief in surgically treated patients. In contrast others have noted that as many as 60% of their patients may be pain free in spite of continuous drinking.[3] To reconcile the apparent different effects of alcohol on pain one can postulate that it is possible that pain not only results from the direct effect of alcohol ingestion but also is related to the functional secretory capacity of the pancreas. In patients with moderate pancreatitis and preserved secretory capacity, alcohol may stimulate secretion and aggravate the pain, whereas in more advanced cases, when most of the parenchyma is replaced by fibrotic tissue, alcohol has less of a stimulatory effect and less impact on the character or frequency of pain.

Stricture and Dilation of the Ducts with Inflammation of the Surrounding Tissue

A direct relationship between pain and ductal strictures and dilations has been accepted for years. When this assumption has been carefully scrutinized, however, several exceptions are noted. For instance, there is no obvious correlation between the morphology of the main, secondary, and tertiary pancreatic ducts as observed by endoscopic retrograde pancreatography (ERP) and the severity of pain.[4] It is not uncommon to find some patients without pancreatic duct abnormalities who experience severe abdominal pain and others with markedly dilated and tortuous ducts who experience minimal or no pain. To illustrate further the unclear relationship between strictures and pain, one study assessed the effect of jejunopancreatic anastomosis on relief of pain and found that all patients (13 out of 13) felt marked relief of pain after surgery, although the anastomosis, as evaluated by ERP, was patent in only four of them.[5]

Pseudocysts

Whenever a pseudocyst is detected and does not resolve spontaneously with conservative management the common experience is that its drainage by either surgical or nonsurgical procedures is usually followed by pain relief.

There are two non-surgical modalities to drain pancreatic pseudocysts.

Endoscopic Drainage

Endoscopic drainage appears to be safe when the cyst is bulging on the posterior wall of the stomach or duodenal lumen. A cystgastrostomy or cystduodenostomy can be performed with the tip of an endoscopic sphincterotome. This approach should be reserved for patients who are high surgical risks and be performed by an experienced endoscopist, since this method may be associated with complications such as bleeding and perforations.[6]

MEDICAL TREATMENT

Percutaneous Aspiration with a Needle Guided by US or CT Scan

Percutaneous aspiration offers the advantage of immediate pain relief, although cysts often recur. Repeated aspiration or drainage through a stent may be needed once the cyst has walled off. The addition of somatostatin in cases with high output may be considered.

Pancreatic Nerve Alterations

Recently Bockman et al studied the fine structure of pancreatic nerves in patients with chronic pancreatitis and found a significant increase in the diameter of the fibers with edema and inflammatory changes. Perhaps of greater importance, these authors found that the protective perineural sheath was destroyed, exposing these nerves to potentially toxic agents (eg, enzymes, kinins) that might cause chemical irritation.[7] Other studies have demonstrated an increase in the amount of neurotransmitters such as calcitonin-gene related peptide and substance P that may be involved in the inflammatory process and the mechanisms of pain.[8] These findings may explain persistence of pain in many patients who do not have ductal abnormalities, pseudocysts, or both.

PRACTICAL APPROACH

When a patient has chronic alcoholic pancreatitis and persistent abdominal pain and possible complications or other causes of abdominal pain have been ruled out, the first step the physician should take is to ensure that the patient is no longer drinking alcohol. This obviously implies an investigation in depth of the causes of alcoholism, interaction with a counselor, and in most cases, referral to a rehabilitation center. In addition a well-balanced diet providing between 2500 and 3000 kcal per day, consisting of 100 to 150 g of protein, 300 to 400 g of carbohydrate, and 70 to 80 g of fat, is indicated. Analgesia can be achieved with increasing doses of acetylsalicylic acid, acetaminophen, nonsteroidal antiinflammatory drugs, and tricyclic antidepressants. Anticholinergics in the usual doses do not seem to provide analgesia in these patients. If pain continues a trial of pancreatic extracts is justified, while at the same time concomitant pathology such as gallstones and peptic ulcer disease are ruled out.

PAIN AND PANCREATIC EXTRACTS

Administration of exogenous pancreatic enzymes, notably proteases, decreases pancreatic enzyme secretion in experimental animals and human subjects.[9] This effect constitutes a normal negative feedback mechanism and involves less cholecystokinin

(CCK) release by the duodenal mucosa because trypsin and other proteases inactivate a CCK-releasing factor (a monitor peptide contained in pancreatic juice and perhaps other secretions).[10] When large quantities of pancreatic proteases are given acutely to patients with chronic pancreatitis, pancreatic secretion is suppressed. When they are given chronically, an amelioration in the intensity of pain is observed in some patients. These were mainly female patients with idiopathic pancreatitis, moderate pancreatic insufficiency and without steatorrhea. Patients with more advanced pancreatitis and exocrine insufficiency, such as those with steatorrhea, did not have similar suppression of pancreatic secretion and had less relief of pain.[9,11] Based on these findings it seems worthwhile to initiate a trial with large doses of pancreatic extracts. In spite of the cost and number of tablets ingested per day, the pain relief observed in some patients is encouraging.

NARCOTICS

When pain is persistent and debilitating, every effort should be made to rule out other causes of failure, such as poor compliance and addiction. The possibility of surgical or endoscopic intervention should be seriously considered. If there is no reasonable option, then analgesia should be provided. The physician must judge, however, the demand and dependence that may develop. About 20% of patients with chronic pancreatitis require narcotics, and addiction may occur in as many as half of them.

Intermediate Narcotics

Intermediate narcotics include: codeine, 15 to 60 mg orally q 4–6 h or parenterally 60 to 120 mg q 4–6 h; oxycodone with aspirin, phenacetin, and caffeine (Percodan) or oxycodone with acetaminophen (Percocet), 5 to 10 mg PO q 4–6 h; propoxyphene (Darvon), 65 mg PO q 3–4 h; pentazocine (Talwin), 50 to 100 mg PO q 4–6 h or parenterally 30 to 60 mg q 4–6 h.

More Potent Narcotics

More potent narcotics include: morphine, 10 mg IM q 4–6 h; meperidine (Demerol), 50 to 100 mg either PO or IM q 4–6 h; hydromorphone (Dilaudid), 1 to 2 mg PO q 3–4 h or 2 mg IM q 4–6 h.

PANCREATIC DENERVATION

An alternative to prevent addiction is to denervate the pancreas by injection of alcohol into the celiac plexus. The procedure is usually performed by skilled anesthesiologists under image-intensifier x-rays with about 25 ml of 50% alcohol injected anterior to the body of the first lumbar vertebra. This method is successful in large numbers of patients with malignancies, and in some cases of chronic pancreatitis relief may be achieved for a few months, although repeated injections may be needed.[12]

ALTERNATIVE TREATMENTS

Attempts have been made to relieve pain by inducing pancreatic atrophy by injecting endoscopically sclerosing solutions or an acrylic glue into the pancreatic duct. Surgical ligature of the main pancreatic duct has also been attempted.[13,14] These new modalities may be considered in selected cases but more experience is needed before they can be recommended.

Management of Malabsorption

Normally the pancreas secretes an amount of enzymes exceeding what is needed to digest a regular meal. Thus, malabsorption does not occur until the enzyme output is reduced by more than 90%. In most cases of chronic alcoholic pancreatitis malabsorption is observed 10 years after the clinical onset. Lipase activity seems to be affected more selectively, and steatorrhea occurs earlier than creatorrhea and carbohydrate malabsorption.

Enzyme Preparations

Most enzyme preparations are extracts of hog pancreas containing a mixture of pancreatic enzymes with variable lipase activity (Table 12.1). Pancreatic enzyme replacement may be started by administering 30,000 to 50,000 units of lipase with each meal. There is no advantage administering the enzymes in several doses throughout the day. It must be understood that it is not possible to completely replace pancreatic function and eliminate steatorrhea. The goal is reduction or elimination of diarrhea, weight gain, and resumption of work. The treatment is life-long, and this should be explained to the patient. In some patients replacement therapy is not successful. This may be due to different reasons.

1. The dosage may be insufficient. Some chronic pancreatitis patients are hyperphagic and ingest higher amounts of fat. Increasing the enzyme doses may solve the problem in these cases. Careful evaluation of the patient response should be made, however, since increasing enzymes is associated with abdominal distension and cramps in some patients. In addition a known complication of enzyme therapy is the development of hyperuricosuria, which could result in clinical manifestations of gout or kidney stones if the doses are increased excessively.

2. Some of the enteric coated preparations are ineffective because of slow gastric emptying of the tablets, capsules, or microspheres, which results in poor mixing

TABLE 12.1. **Enzyme Preparations: Potency as Determined by Lipase Content**

Preparation	Lipase Content (U/Tablet or Capsule)
Ilozyme (nonenteric tablet)	11,000
Viokase (tablets)	8000
(powder, 1/4 tsp)	16,800
Cotazym (capsules)	8000
(enteric coated spheres)	5000
Ku-zyme HP (capsules)	8000
Pancrease (enteric coated microspheres)	4000
Pancrease MT4 (enteric coated microtabs)	4000
Pancrease MT10	10,000
Pancrease MT16	16,000
Pancrex V Forte (tablets)	5600
Zymase (enteric coated spheres)	10,000
Entolase (enteric coated capsules)	4000
Pancreatin (enteric coated microspheres)	7700
Entolase HP (enteric coated microbeads)	8000
Creon (enteric coated microspheres)	8000

Possible side effects: nausea, vomiting, diarrhea, abdominal cramps, hyperuricosuria, and hyperuricemia.

of the enzymes with the meal in the intestine. The opposite situation may occur in patients who have had gastric surgery with accelerated gastric emptying. Administration of pancreatic extracts in powder form appears to have better results in these cases.

3. Enzymes in general, and lipase in particular, can be inactivated in the stomach by the acid medium and pepsin. The acidic pH of the duodenum caused by the impaired bicarbonate secretion affects the lipase activity and precipitates bile acids. There are acid-stable lipases in the von Ebner glands and in the gastric mucosa, and interesting studies are being done using a fungal lipase which is resistant to acid pH, does not require co-lipase, and is greatly potentiated by bile salts.[15] Preparations containing this acid lipase are not yet available. The gastric acidity factor can be corrected by administration of enteric coated preparations, or by the use of enzyme extracts with concomitant administration of antacids or acid suppression with H_2-receptor antagonists or proton pump inhibitors. Some of the most common antacids contain mixtures of magnesium–aluminum hydroxide that raise intragastric pH, particularly when given shortly after meals, but tend to form soaps in the intestine where fatty acids become free after hydrolysis by lipase. Magnesium-containing antacids also may aggravate diarrhea. For these reasons in some patients the addition of sodium bicarbonate is preferred, although the consequences of giving high amounts of sodium should be considered in patients with concomitant hypertension, congestive heart disease, or ascites. The experiences with cimetidine or other H_2-receptor antagonists are not uniformly positive

and the use of newer agents like omeprazole needs further clinical evaluation. An alternative therapeutic possibility is to administer enzymes in microspheres coated with a film that dissolves in alkaline medium. This preparation should be given during meals.[16]

4. Lipase may be destroyed by proteolysis in the intestine. It has been observed that lipase activity decreases in vitro in duodenal juice containing proteases.[17] In healthy subjects this effect does not represent a serious problem because lipase is secreted in large amounts, but it may become critical when there is marked insufficiency. Adding soybean trypsin inhibitor to pancreatic extracts may reduce the degree of steatorrhea. If, after all the corrections, there is no positive response, the diagnosis of chronic pancreatitis should be reconsidered or therapy evaluated with one of the tubeless tests.

Management of Diabetes

Diabetes mellitus occurs late in the course of chronic pancreatitis and its incidence seems to be higher (70%) in calcified compared with noncalcified forms (30%). Its presentation seems to be shorter from the time of disease onset in alcoholic pancreatitis compared with pancreatitis related to other causes. Diabetes in pancreatitis usually is moderate and complications occur rarely, with the exception of peripheral neuropathy in alcoholics, in whom both diabetes and alcoholism may certainly contribute. Symptoms are related to exaggerated and prolonged postprandial or fasting hyperglycemia. When diabetic patients have steatorrhea the diagnosis of pancreatitis should always be considered in the differential diagnosis. Diabetes may be brittle and hypoglycemic episodes probably occur because it is difficult for alcoholics to follow a diet strictly, and also because pancreatitis patients seem to have abnormal glucagon release.[18] Thus, if insulin is given, the doses should be moderate and symptoms of hypoglycemia should be explained to the patient and relatives, so they can act promptly should it occur.

SURGERY FOR PAIN IN CHRONIC PANCREATITIS

Indications

The indications for surgery for pain relief in patients with chronic pancreatitis are difficult to state precisely. In general, when the pain interferes substantially with the quality of life, surgery should be considered. Important issues to consider include effects on health and well-being such as weight loss and poor nutritional status, need for frequent hospitalization, inability to maintain employment, psychiatric manifestations (usually depression), deterioration of family life, and narcotic addiction.

All patients who are evaluated for possible surgical intervention should undergo an abdominal CT scan and usually an endoscopic retrograde cholangiopancreatography (ERCP) to demonstrate ductal anatomy.[19] In addition to the standard preoperative assessment for a major abdominal procedure, arteriography may be helpful for those in whom pancreatic resection is being considered. Psychiatric evaluation is also appropriate in many patients. These studies are necessary to provide information about the type of surgical procedure indicated, as well as determining whether a procedure is appropriate at all. Although decisions for surgery are always the result of a risk-versus-benefit assessment, this is particularly so in this group of patients. Thus, a major pancreatic resection is contraindicated in alcoholic patients who are addicted to narcotics because these patients cannot handle responsibly the diabetic state that often ensues. A pancreaticojejunostomy may be perfectly safe and appropriate in such a patient, however, because this operation does not create diabetes.

Operations to relieve pain in patients with chronic pancreatitis take one of two forms. The first are the so-called drainage operations, which attempt to drain more adequately a dilated ductal system.[20,21] The second are the pancreatic resection operations, which remove diseased pancreatic tissue, usually in situations where the pancreatic ducts are normal or narrowed in size.[22-24] Sphincterotomy or sphincteroplasty of the sphincter of Oddi is not appropriate in the treatment of pain in patients with this disease.

Drainage Procedures

The main pancreatic duct has a normal diameter of approximately 4 to 5 mm in the head, 3 to 4 mm in the body, and 2 to 3 mm in the tail of the gland. When the diameter in the head and body increases to 7 to 8 mm or larger, a pancreaticojejunostomy is technically feasible and is likely to be effective. The pancreatic duct is opened up longitudinally from the head of the pancreas near the duodenum well into the tail of the gland (Fig. 12.1). Any calcifications that may be present are removed, and the open duct is anastomosed to a defunctionalized limb of jejunum. If the operation is done in a pancreas with a normally sized duct, both short-term and long-term results are poor, perhaps because the anastomosis strictures close in most cases.[20,21]

This lateral pancreaticojejunostomy is currently the preferred operation when the duct is dilated. The operative mortality rate is low (<4%). There is no significant short-term or long-term morbidity. Diabetes does not result from the operation, although a number of patients will eventually require insulin since the destruction of the pancreas continues. It provides pain relief in about 80% of patients for the first few years. After 5 years, however, some authors find that only about 50% are still free of pain. Others have been more optimistic, and reported that two thirds to three fourths of patients remain free of pain up to 6 years.[22,25] Although pancreatic enzymes can now empty freely through the pancreaticojejunostomy (Fig. 12.2), there is rarely any clinical improvement in the degree of malabsorption. Nevertheless, patients may gain weight because eating no longer produces pain, and they eat more. In some patients recurrence of pain may be due to stenosis of the pancreaticojejunal anastomosis, which can be proved by ERCP.[20] Then reconstruction of the anastomosis may be beneficial. In the majority of cases, there is no apparent cause for the recurrence

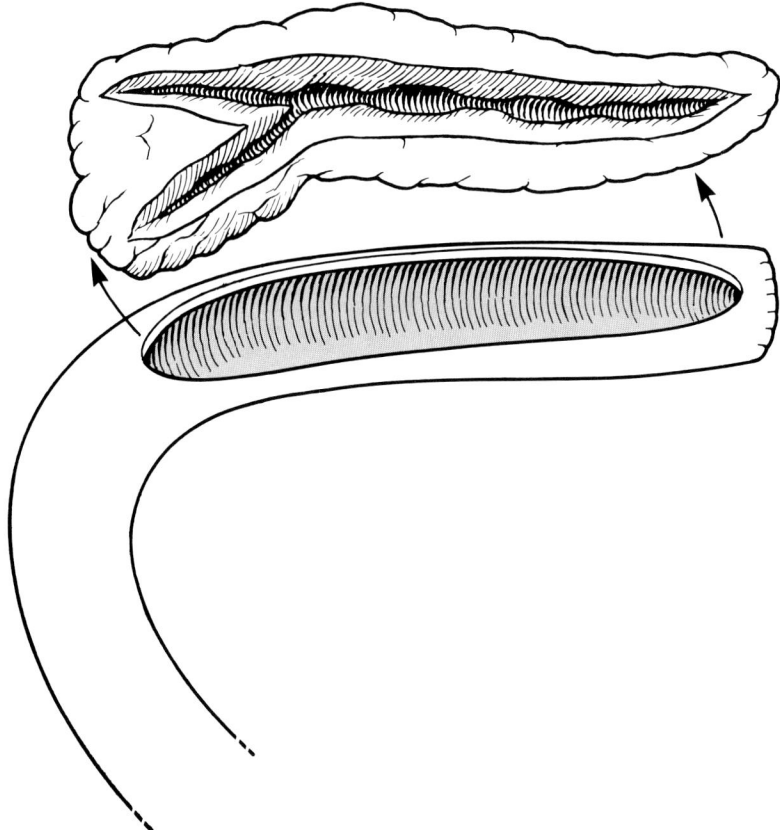

FIGURE 12.1. The pancreatic duct has been opened throughout the entire length of the pancreas. A roux-en-y limb of jejunum is prepared for anastomosis to the cut duct. The opening in the jejunum is tailored to fit in each case.

of pain, and other forms of treatment, including pancreatic resection, must be considered.

Pancreatic Resections

Pancreatic resection (pancreaticoduodenectomy, pylorus-preserving pancreaticoduodenectomy, pancreatic head resection, 95% pancreatectomy, distal pancreatectomy) should be considered for pain relief when the pancreatic duct is narrow or normal in diameter, when a previous pancreaticojejunostomy has failed, or when the pathologic changes in the pancreas particularly involve one part of the gland and the rest is less diseased.[26,27]

For example, when the head of the pancreas is especially thickened, compresses the bile duct, or contains multiple cysts and calcifications, a Whipple pancreaticoduo-

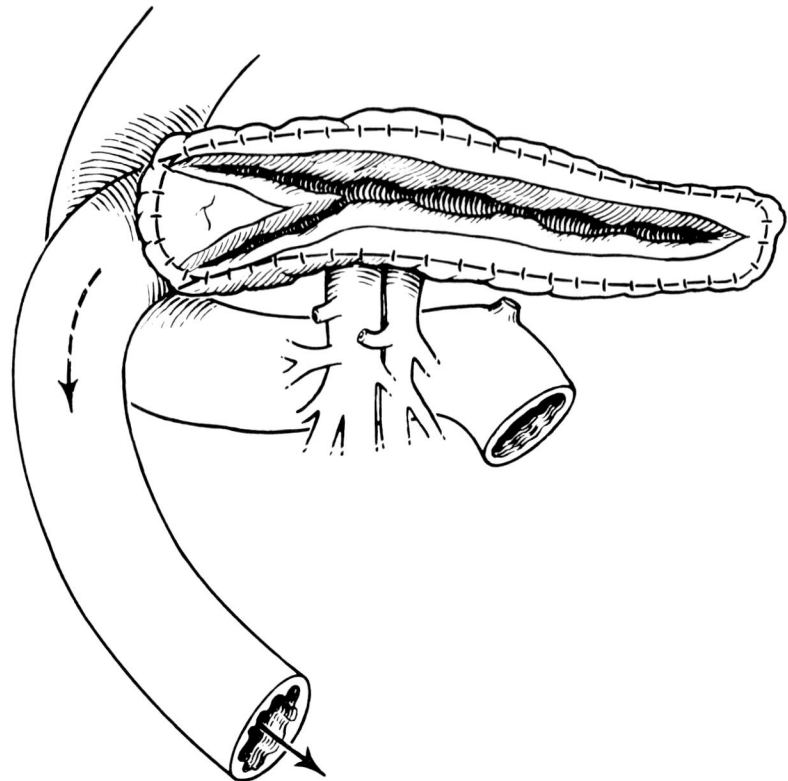

FIGURE 12.2. The jejunum has been anastomosed to the opened pancreatic duct. This relieves the ductal obstruction, decompresses the pancreatic tissue, and allows the pancreatic juice to empty freely into the gastrointestinal tract.

denectomy may be considered. This is the operation that is usually done for pancreatic cancer, but it is also effective for pain relief in patients with chronic pancreatitis. A modification of this operation is the pancreaticoduodenectomy with preservation of the stomach and pylorus. The theoretical advantage of the latter is that it preserves gastric function and avoids some of the nutritional disturbances that may follow the standard pancreaticoduodenectomy. The few comparisons that have been made so far have failed to prove that preservation of the distal stomach and pylorus confers significant benefit, however.[28] The postoperative recovery is complicated by delayed gastric emptying in a significant number of patients, but this resolves eventually.

New operations have been described in which the head of the pancreas is resected and the entire stomach and duodenum are preserved.[29,30] The body and tail of the pancreas as well as a thin rim of pancreatic tissue in the C loop of the duodenum also remain. The theoretical advantages of the procedure include preservation of gastroduodenal and biliary continuity and function and, because most of the pancreas is preserved, a low likelihood of the development of diabetes. The procedure has been done in patients in whom most of the pathologic changes involved the head of the pancreas, with duodenal compression in about half, common bile duct compression in two thirds, and compression of the portal vein in one quarter of the cases. Although the results appear promising both from the point of preservation of endocrine function and the relief of pain (80% at 3.5 years), longer follow-up study and confirmation of these results in other centers will be important.

Ninety-five percent distal pancreatectomy entails the removal of the spleen and all of the pancreas except for a thin rim of tissue that lies within the C loop of the duodenum. Because the spleen is sacrificed and all of the patients require insulin after this operation, it is not done frequently. Nevertheless if the entire pancreas is uniformly and severely diseased, and especially if lesser operations have failed to provide relief, it may be considered. Total pancreatectomy is rarely done today because of the uniform requirement for insulin and the significant alterations in digestive and absorptive functions that follow. The 95% pancreatectomy, which preserves normal gastrointestinal and biliary continuity, is often preferred in situations where such a major resection is indicated.

Distal pancreatectomy is an imprecise term that describes resection of variable amounts of the tail or body and tail of the pancreas, in which the head of the gland is preserved. In most instances a splenectomy is also part of the pancreatic resection, even if the splenic vein is patent. This is because of the difficulty often encountered in separating the splenic vein from the adherent pancreatic parenchyma.

The operative mortality rates for pancreaticoduodenectomy and subtotal resections of the pancreas vary between 5% and 10%. In general a pancreaticoduodenectomy can be performed by experienced surgeons with a mortality rate of about 5%. Pain is relieved in about 80% of the patients in the first several years after the operation. Unlike patients who have undergone longitudinal pancreaticojejunostomy, this initial good result is more likely to be permanent after resection.

References

1. Hajnal F, Flores MC, Radley S, et al. Effect of alcohol and alcoholic beverages on meal-stimulated pancreatic secretion in humans. *Gastroenterology* 1990;98:191–196.
2. Trapell JE. Chronic relapsing pancreatitis: a review of 64 cases. *Br J Surg* 1979;66:471–475.
3. Ink O, Labayle D, Buffet C, et al. Pancreatite chronique alcoolique: relation de la douleur avec le sevrage et la chirurgie pancreatique. *Gastroenterol Clin Biol* 1984;8:419–425.
4. Bornman PC, Marks IN, Girdwood AH, et al. Is pancreatic duct obstruction or stricture a major cause of pain in calcific pancreatitis? *Br J Surg* 1980;67:425–428.
5. Kugelberg CA, Wehlin L, Arnsjo B, et al. Endoscopic pancreatography in evaluating results of pancreatic-jejunostomy. *Gut* 1976;17:267–274.
6. Sahel J, Liguory C. Endoscopic treatment of pancreatic cysts: preliminary results. *Gastroenterology* 1984;86:1227. (Abstract.)
7. Bockman DE, Buchler M, Malfertheiner P, et al. Analysis of nerves in chronic pancreatitis. *Gastroenterology* 1988;94:1459–1469.
8. Buchler M, Weihe E, Malfertheiner P, et al. Neurotransmitters in nerves in chronic pancreatitis. *Pancreas* 1988;3:592.
9. Slaff J, Jacabson D, Tillman CR, et al. Protease-specific suppression of pancreatic exocrine secretion. *Gastroenterology* 1984;87:44–52.

10. Iwai K, Fushiki T, Fukuoka S. Pancreatic enzyme secretion mediated by novel peptide: monitor peptide hypothesis. *Pancreas* 1988;3:720–728.
11. Isaksson F, Ihse I. Pain reduction by an oral pancreatic enzyme preparation in chronic pancreatitis. *Dig Dis Sci* 1983;28:97–102.
12. Heving JWC, Borven-Wright M, Areling W, et al. Coeliac plexus block for pain in pancreatic cancer and chronic pancreatitis. *Br J Surg* 1983;70:730–732.
13. Hutson DG, Levi JU, Livingstone A, et al. Pancreatic duct ligation in the therapy of chronic pancreatitis. *Am Surg* 1979;45:449–452.
14. Little JM, Stephen M, Hogg J. Duct obstruction with an acrylate glue for treatment of chronic alcoholic pancreatitis. *Lancet* 1979;2:557–558.
15. Schneider MU, Knoll-Ruzicka MC, Domschke S, et al. Pancreatic enzyme replacement therapy: comparative effects of conventional and enteric coated microspheric pancreatic and acid stable fungal enzymes preparation on steatorrhea in chronic pancreatitis. *Hepatogastroenterology* 1985;32:97–102.
16. Ihse I, Lilja P, Lunquist I. Intestinal concentrations of pancreatic enzymes following pancreatic replacement therapy. *Scand J Gastroenterol* 1980;15:137–144.
17. Thiruvengadam R, DiMagno EP. Inactivation of human lipase by proteases. *Am J Physiol* 1988;255:G476–G481.
18. Marks IN, Bank S, Vinik AI. Clinical and hormonal aspects of pancreatic diabetes. *Am J Gastroenterol* 1975;64:13–22.
19. Reber H. Chronic pancreatitis: etiology, diagnosis and pathology. In: Howard JM, Jordan GL, Reber HA, eds. *Surgical Diseases of the Pancreas*. Philadelphia: Lea & Febiger, 1987: 475–495.
20. Prinz RA, Greenlee HB. Pancreatic duct drainage in 100 patients with chronic pancreatitis. *Ann Surg* 1981;194:313–320.
21. Ihse I, Lankisch PG. Treatment of chronic pancreatitis—current status. *Acta Chir Scand* 1988;154:553–558.
22. Bradley EL. Long-term results of pancreatojejunostomy in patients with chronic pancreatitis. *Am J Surg* 1987;153:207–213.
23. Frey CF, Child CG, Fry WF. Pancreatectomy for chronic pancreatitis. *Ann Surg* 1976; 184:403–413.
24. Sarles J-C, Nacchiero M, Garani F, et al. Surgical treatment of chronic pancreatitis: report of 134 cases treated by resection or drainage. *Am J Surg* 1982;144:317–321.
25. Sato T, Miyashita E, Matsuno S, et al. The role of surgical treatment for chronic pancreatitis. *Ann Surg* 1986;203:266–271.
26. Keith RG, Saibil FG, Sheppard RH. Treatment of chronic alcoholic pancreatitis by pancreatic resection. *Am J Surg* 1989;157:156–162.
27. Moossa AR. Surgical treatment of chronic pancreatitis: an overview. *Br J Surg* 1987; 74:661–667.
28. Fink A, DeSouza LR, Mayer J, et al. Long-term evaluation of pylorus preservation during pancreaticoduodenectomy. *World J Surg* 1988;12:663.
29. Beger HG, Krautzberger W, Bittner R. Duodenum preserving resection of the head of the pancreas in patients with severe chronic pancreatitis. *Surgery* 1985;97:467.
30. Frey CF, Smith GJ. Description and rationale of a new operation for chronic pancreatitis. *Pancreas* 1987;2:701–707.

Chapter 13

Pancreatic Disease in Infants and Children

JOEL W. ADELSON

In this chapter the major diseases of the exocrine pancreas in the pediatric population will be briefly described. A number of these illnesses, for example, acute pancreatitis, overlap in both their pathophysiology and clinical characteristics with the same illness in the adult population. In such cases the reader is referred to more complete material on the subject that appears elsewhere in this volume (see Chapters 3, 4 and 5). Features of pancreatic disease more specific to infants and children are highlighted here. Several volumes on pediatric gastroenterology contain fairly complete reviews of the material summarized here.[1-3] The interested reader should consult these before making significant decisions based on the summary material presented in this chapter only.

CONGENITAL ABERRATIONS OF PANCREATIC MORPHOLOGY

Annular Pancreas

Annular pancreas occurs as a result of aberrant embryogenic formation at the head of the pancreas, and ultimately results in a portion of the gland completely encircling the descending portion of the duodenum. The anomaly causes a partial or complete block of the intestine with obstruction at the duodenal level and usually presents acutely in early infancy with signs of upper gastrointestinal tract obstruction. Since varying degrees of duodenal atresia accompany the annular pancreas, it always presents in early infancy when obstruction is severe. Variations that are less obstructive may be seen later or may never become clinically evident. Annular pancreas appears to result from partially understood anomalous variations in development of the dorsal or ventral pancreatic anlagae and ducts; at surgery a good deal of variability is found in the resultant drainage of the gland. A typical radiographic sign in infants is distention caused by air of both the stomach and duodenum proximal to the obstruction seen on a plain film of the abdomen; this sign is known as the "double bubble," and is also seen in duodenal atresia. Treatment is usually by surgical bypass of the annulus, since attempts to divide the encircling ring may create future difficulties with the outlet of the common duct into the duodenum. The entity is found with increased frequency in Down's syndrome.

CASE PRESENTATION

>A 3-day-old male infant was born to a 32-year-old gravida two, para one woman at 39 weeks gestation following an uncomplicated pregnancy. The infant was breast fed, but began to vomit forcefully within hours of birth. An initial examination and survey of the complete blood count (CBC), electrolytes, and glucose at 12 hours showed modest dehydration and a glucose of 38. Intravenous glucose and electrolytes were administered, and the infant was transferred to a pediatric center, where initial investigation included a plain film of the abdomen that revealed a "double bubble" sign of air in the stomach and duodenum, with little air in the distal bowel. At surgery, annular pancreas and duodenal obstruction with partial atresia were found. A gastrojejunostomy was performed. The postoperative course was uneventful and the child was discharged at 16 days of age.

Pancreas divisum occurs in both children and adults and may be diagnosed by endoscopic retrograde cholangiopancreatography (ERCP) in a small fraction of cases and seems to be associated with acute or relapsing pancreatitis. The association between clinical pancreatic disease and this anatomic variation, which leads to separate drainage from the dorsal and ventral pancreatic anlagae, is not clear. Two papillae are found in these patients; it has been proposed that dysfunction of the accessory papilla is also required for pancreatitis to develop. The anomaly frequently causes no clinical problems and is only an incidental finding on autopsy; there are no specific pediatric features to this entity.

Congenital pancreatic aplasia or hypoplasia occur as both partial and total lack of development of the exocrine gland, with accompanying paucity of endocrine tissue function. Both aplasia and hypoplasia are exceedingly rare. The anomaly exhibits the physiologic and clinical features of total pancreatic insufficiency from more common causes such as cystic fibrosis, discussed below, but it may be differentiated from cystic fibrosis in that sweat chloride testing is normal, and it does not exhibit the multiple hematologic, bony, and immunologic features of the Shwachman-Diamond syndrome.

Other congenital anomalies include variations with respect to the location and formation of the junction of the bile and pancreatic ducts. Anomalies in this area may result in choledochal cyst formation with consequent obstruction of hepatobiliary outflow. Such anomalies are discovered occasionally during the neonatal period. Although they involve the pancreas, they are found more frequently as a cause of obstructive jaundice in the neonate than as a cause of any problem directly referable to the pancreas.

As in adults, heterotopic pancreatic tissue or "pancreatic rests" are found in children at various upper gastrointestinal tract locations as rare causes of obstruction, bleeding, and intussusception. An occasional pancreatic rest may mimic pyloric stenosis.

As in adults, various forms of primary cystic structures occur in children, at times due to duplication of the intestine in the region near the pancreas, and at other times intrinsic to the gland itself, and the consequent ductular obstruction causes the consequent development of one of several forms of pancreatitis.

EXOCRINE FUNCTIONAL PANCREATIC INSUFFICIENCY IN THE PEDIATRIC POPULATION

Cystic Fibrosis

Two illnesses, cystic fibrosis and the Shwachman-Diamond syndrome, both of which are inherited in an autosomal recessive pattern, may present with severe failure to thrive in infancy and childhood. Cystic fibrosis is an important genetic illness that occurs in all races, but primarily in whites, and presents with a broad spectrum of degrees of exocrine pancreatic insufficiency, most commonly during infancy and early childhood.[3] In about 85% of cases, failure to secrete pancreatic digestive enzymes is a prominent feature from the time of first diagnosis. Since exocrine pancreatic insufficiency becomes clinically manifested only when most of pancreatic function is lost (80% to 90% of total pancreatic capacity must be diminished before clinical symptoms are noted) a significant degree of loss of pancreatic function may occur and be tolerated without obvious clinical consequences before the final development of steatorrhea and failure-to-thrive.

Although the gene frequency varies widely among different populations, among North American whites the carrier rate is very high, with about one in 25.5 persons carrying the recessive allele as a heterozygote. Since most cystic fibrosis carriers have until now been unaware of their carrier state, about one in 650 couples have both parents as carriers ($1/25.5 \times 1/25.5 = 1/650$), and this in turn leads to a theoretical birth rate of about one in 2500 births, since one in four of the offspring will receive both defective alleles. Among couples with one heterozygote carrier, half the children will be carriers. Since the discovery of the gene carrying the defect, a degree of heterogeneity has been found among the alleles; this will complicate the analysis of the carrier state (4).

Cystic fibrosis is due to a specific deletion in a gene, which specifies a structural feature of a protein that, when modeled for its structure, was found to probably form a channel responsible for the movement of chloride ions across the external cell membrane of various types of epithelial tissues. The gene occurs on the long arm of chromosome 7 in the human genome.[5-7] The gene product has not yet been directly or extensively characterized. The chloride channel has probably been best characterized thus far in the sweat gland and respiratory epithelium. The channel appears to be fairly ubiquitous throughout most epithelial tissues, including the ductular system of the exocrine pancreas, where it is involved in the secretion of chloride, water, and possibly bicarbonate into the exocrine pancreatic fluid.

The defective chloride channel in the different tissues has been implicated to varying degrees in the pathophysiologic mechanisms underlying the illness. In the sweat gland in healthy individuals, the orientation of the channel appears to function to allow transport of earlier secreted chloride out of the ductal lumen (resorption); thus, defective function of the channel in cystic fibrosis results in excess chloride remaining in the sweat at the point of secretion on the skin. This anomaly in chloride resorption from sweat currently forms the basis for the most widely recognized and employed method of diagnosis, in which sweat is collected and analyzed for its chloride content. A clearly elevated sweat chloride, in the absence of confounding factors such as severe malnutrition, is considered diagnostic of the disease. With the advent of genetic analysis for the disease and direct identification of the anomalous gene, it might be expected that the sweat test will be replaced by a DNA hybridization method applicable to both prenatal and postnatal diagnosis based on recognition of the aberrant gene sequence in a suitable tissue or blood sample. Such a probe capable of heterozygote analysis has been reported (4). This raises the possibility of general screening programs, available to all or designated portions of the population. It is to be hoped that any use of such probes will occur in populations that have been well informed; cystic fibrosis causes fear among prospective parents, and erroneous ideas, such as if one parent is a carrier the couple is at risk, may irrationally affect childbearing decisions.

The specific defect caused by the gene as expressed in the exocrine pancreas has been only partially characterized. Again, and as predicted,[8] it appears to be attributable to the defective chloride channel. It has been shown that stimulation of exocrine pancreatic secretion from infants and children with cystic fibrosis results in a failure of enzyme secretion, which in turn is *secondary* to a greatly diminished fluid output by the gland.[9] Even in patients in whom exocrine enzyme secretion is partially but not totally diminished, the defect in fluid secretion can be directly demonstrated by pancreatic stimulation testing.[10] It is presumed that the failure of pancreatic fluid secretion eventually results in an inability to dissolve and transport secreted digestive enzymes out of the acinar lumen and ductular system of the pancreas and into the digestive tract proper. The secreted enzymes are therefore left inspissated in the uppermost small caliber pancreatic ducts, where they lead to slow and permanent destruction of the pancreatic tissue. The process is occasionally accompanied by frank pancreatitis. Most often, however, the process of loss of pancreatic function is indolent, and exocrine pancreatic insufficiency develops silently during the prenatal period and continues after birth. It is not clear that the inspissated enzymes entirely account for the overall failure of enzyme secretion. At birth, some infants already exhibit fully developed pancreatic insufficiency, contributing to an inability to digest meconium (the content of the prenatal gut); such infants are born with a congenitally-obstructed intestine due to "meconium ileus." Others will present in early, middle, or later infancy, or at anytime throughout childhood with steatorrhea and failure-to-thrive. Although pancreatic insufficiency can manifest at any time from infancy to adulthood, it usually occurs in the first few years of life. At times the endocrine pancreas can become involved in the pathologic process as well, with resultant hypoinsulinemia and poor glucose tolerance.

Examination of the patient presenting with cystic fibrosis reveals varying degrees of failure-to-thrive and frank clinical wasting with or without edema, and often with pneumonia or otherwise abnormal chest films. Diarrhea is frequent but not universal; often the stools are semiformed but bulky, float in the toilet basin, and are visibly oily. In infancy the abnormal stools may not be obvious. Laboratory examination will show excess fat in the stool; hypoproteinemia, hypoalbuminemia, anemia, fat-soluble vitamin deficiencies, and essential fatty acid deficiency may occur. The diagnosis of cystic fibrosis should be strongly suspected and actively sought in all infants with meconium ileus. The diagnosis should be considered within the differential diagnosis of infants and children with failure-to-thrive. Failure-to-thrive implies a wide differential diagnostic spectrum, however, with many causes including malabsorption due to other diseases, and investigation of such patients yields only a small minority with cystic fibrosis. As described above, pancreatic insufficiency is not universally found in all newly diagnosed patients with cystic fibrosis, and a significant number of patients are diagnosed because of the prominence of other symptoms of the disease, usually respiratory problems.

In older patients pancreatic insufficiency combined with the presence of thick intestinal secretions may lead to a complex of systems of abdominal pain with subacute obstruction of the small bowel. This complex, known as "meconium ileus equivalent," appears to be most prominent in children who are approaching adolescence, and thereafter.

Cystic fibrosis has a profound effect on the respiratory tract, leading to secretion of thickened mucus with repeated respiratory infections, chronic lung disease, and ultimately pulmonary failure with cor pulmonale. As many as 15% of patients exhibit respiratory problems in the absence of pancreatic insufficiency. Again, the infant or child with ongoing chronic respiratory problems should be considered for sweat testing for cystic fibrosis if other diagnoses are not made. In general, however, cystic fibrosis is typically manifested in infancy and early childhood by predominance of symptoms due to pancreatic insufficiency, with respiratory symptoms gradually becoming the predominant clinical feature later in the course of the disease. Cystic fibrosis also clinically affects numerous other organs beyond the pancreas and lungs, including the liver and biliary tract, intestine, and testes.

Treatment of the pancreatic manifestations of cystic fibrosis is directed at restoring the digestive hydrolytic capacity by replacement of deficient pancreatic secretion with orally-administered digestive enzymes. Numerous preparations of enzymes are available in either powder form, capsules, or enteric-coated microspheres that are consumed either in capsules or sprinkled over food. Problems with the administration of active enzymes renders it nearly impossible to restore digestive capacity to the normal range. No matter how much enzyme is taken, some degree of steatorrhea almost invariably remains, and in older patients 20 to 30 of some preparations capsules must be consumed through a meal. Improvements in steatorrhea or fat wasting are highly desirable in cystic fibrosis patients, since this is the major route of caloric loss leading to malnutrition. Attention should be paid to correcting steatorrhea by using enzyme preparations in sufficient quantity—a trial and error process—and by considering the enzyme activity available in the preparation employed, especially the lipase. Some patients may benefit to a degree by diminution of gastric acid production by H_2 blockers, which partially protect the administered enzyme preparation against inactivation in the stomach. Enteric-coated enzyme preparations serve a similar purpose.

Much attention has been paid to the importance of maintenance of as high an overall nutritional status as possible in patients with cystic fibrosis. Patients with cystic fibrosis have increased work of breathing, and must also frequently fight pulmonary infections, both at great caloric expense. This creates a caloric deficiency that can be especially difficult to rectify in the setting of pancreatic insufficiency. When these additional factors are combined with the well-known psychologically depressive effects of illness and malnutrition on appetite and intake, a picture of an ill, depressed, malnourished, and anorexic patient frequently emerges. There is a strong suspicion that both respiratory muscle function and effort will deteriorate more rapidly in the presence of poor nutritional status. Approaches to improved nutrition are multiple. At all ages, administration of medium chain triglycerides (MCT) as a supplement to other caloric sources may be considered; these lipids are less dependent on pancreatic lipase and the lymphatic system for digestion and absorption. Infant formulas containing MCT oil and prehydrolysed peptides are available; for the older patients, the oil may be used as a base for cooking and added to various foods. Fat-soluble vitamin supplementation is especially important; vitamin E deficiency has received much attention and an oral preparation of alpha tocopheryl polyethylene glycol succinate has been shown to be well absorbed.[11] In all patients, generalized dietary supplementation by the voluntary oral route, accompanied by sufficient enzymes, as well as continuous enteral alimentation through a nasogastric tube at night in the home, gastrostomy feeding, and total parenteral nutrition during periods of hospitalization or at home are all available as therapeutic modalities. Aggressive prevention and treatment of the nutritional deficits intrinsic to cystic fibrosis are necessary.

Patients with the suspected or confirmed diagnosis of cystic fibrosis should be referred to, and be followed on an ongoing basis in, a center with a specialized and up-to-date program capable of dealing with the multiple pancreatic, respiratory, and other complications of this serious illness. The discovery of the molecular basis of the illness will have an immediate impact at the clinical level on diagnostic methods, but changes in treatment will be delayed until pharmacologic or genetic approaches to ameliorating the probable chloride channel defect can be developed. This does not appear to be a simple problem.

CASE PRESENTATION

> A 4-month-old female was admitted to a pediatric center for investigation of failure-to-thrive. She was born to a gravida one, para zero, 28-year-old woman after a normal pregnancy and delivery. The birth weight was 3.2 kg. and the infant was fed by breast, but after 10 days appeared hungry and irritable. At 2 months, she was changed to a soy protein-based formula. By 4 months, she weighed only 3.8 kg. and was described as irritable and somewhat lethargic. The stools were somewhat bulky and frequent, but diarrhea was not apparent. At admission, the child was found to be moderately edematous and pale, with a poor muscle mass. Laboratory results showed an abnormal chest film, anemia, hypoalbuminemia, a prolonged clotting time, and a markedly elevated sweat chloride. The initial manifestations of cystic fibrosis in infancy with failure-to-thrive, edema, and anemia are characteristic of one of the forms of the disease. Edema is by no means frequent, however, and can be the cause of a false negative sweat test.

The Shwachman-Diamond syndrome, another autosomal recessive disease, is a rare illness that, like cystic fibrosis, results in exocrine pancreatic insufficiency. Interestingly, the pathophysiology of this illness features a direct failure of enzyme secretion

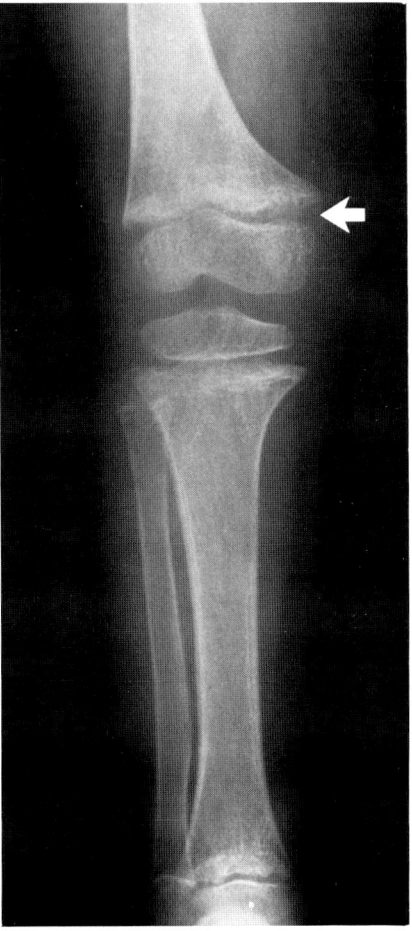

FIGURE 13.1. Shortening of long bones with flaring and irregularity of the metaphyses in a 10.5-year-old girl with the metaphysical dysostosis and dwarfism characteristic of many cases of Shwachman-Diamond syndrome (Courtesy of Michael T. Wallach, MD).

due to replacement of the acinar tissue with fatty material, whereas preservation of the ductular system leads to relatively normal fluid and electrolyte secretion. The Shwachman-Diamond syndrome was discovered primarily as a result of identifying children with pancreatic insufficiency who had normal sweat tests, and the syndrome has proven to be distinct from cystic fibrosis. It is much rarer, and on a primary basis is characterized by a variable spectrum of manifestations. All patients have pancreatic insufficiency, and most have abnormalities in immune function, cyclic or permanent neutropenia, congenital short stature, and a bony abnormality called metaphyseal dysostosis (Fig. 13.1). Congenital short stature is not secondary to nutritional insufficiency, so restoration of the latter will not entirely rectify the short stature, but the growth-inhibiting effects of the nutritional deprivation due to pancreatic insufficiency should be treated vigorously. The diagnosis can be a difficult one; duodenal intubation with pancreatic stimulation is ultimately required, thereby proving lack of enzyme secretion. In addition, a normal sweat test, and establishment of the neutropenia are required. The clinical course appears variable; some patients have severe infections in early childhood due to the immune deficiency, others exhibit a degree of mental retardation, and others tolerate the disease well. The steatorrhea of infancy caused by the pancreatic insufficiency that occurs in this disease may be ameliorated later in the course of this illness. The mechanism of such amelioration is unknown.

PANCREATITIS IN CHILDREN

Pancreatitis occurs in the pediatric population far less frequently than in the adult population, and the major causes are skewed in a different direction. Without a major contribution from alcohol abuse and with only rare cases based on cholelithiasis, the known causes in children are distributed mainly among viral infections, trauma, and drugs. Half of all cases are idiopathic in origin. Viruses are the main specific cause; in addition to mumps several other viruses have been found to be associated with acute pancreatitis. Physical trauma may occasionally cause injury to the exocrine pancreas resulting in acute pancreatitis. Accidents such as a child being kicked in the abdomen or falling over the handlebars of a bicycle, as well as trauma due to child abuse, are known to occasionally cause acute pancreatitis. At times the original cause may be unapparent, since the pancreatic inflammation may begin some days after a minor-appearing injury. As in adults, steroid medication may predispose to acute pancreatitis. Pancreatitis has also been reported in association with a number of cases of Reye syndrome.

As in adults, the classic clinical manifestation has severe pain and vomiting; babies do not localize or verbalize the source of their pain. The diagnosis of acute or chronic pancreatitis differs little from that of adults, with the same considerations of hyperamylasemia, decreased renal clearance of amylase due to other diseases, and the rapid clearance of serum amylase with a longer persistence of elevated serum lipase levels. Generally a demonstration of clearly elevated amylase and lipase levels will suffice for diagnosis. One particular pediatric feature of pancreatitis is the relatively easy visualization of the pancreas on ultrasonography in children compared with adults; dilation of the main pancreatic duct is the most useful diagnostic feature.[12] There are also alterations in pancreatic echodensity; the normal gland, in contrast, is equal in density to the liver). The treatment of pancreatitis in children differs little from adult management of the illness, with the exception that pediatricians and pediatric intensivists have to pay careful attention to fluid and electrolytes on a weight-adjusted basis that considers the small size of the patient. Bowel rest; avoidance of pancreatic stimulation, as discussed elsewhere in this volume; and attention to alternative routes of nutrition are important for the management of the illness. As in adults, pseudocyst formation is a well-known sequel. In recent years ERCP examination of the pancreas has been applied to younger children. In some centers not even infants are exempt from the procedure; however, it should probably be

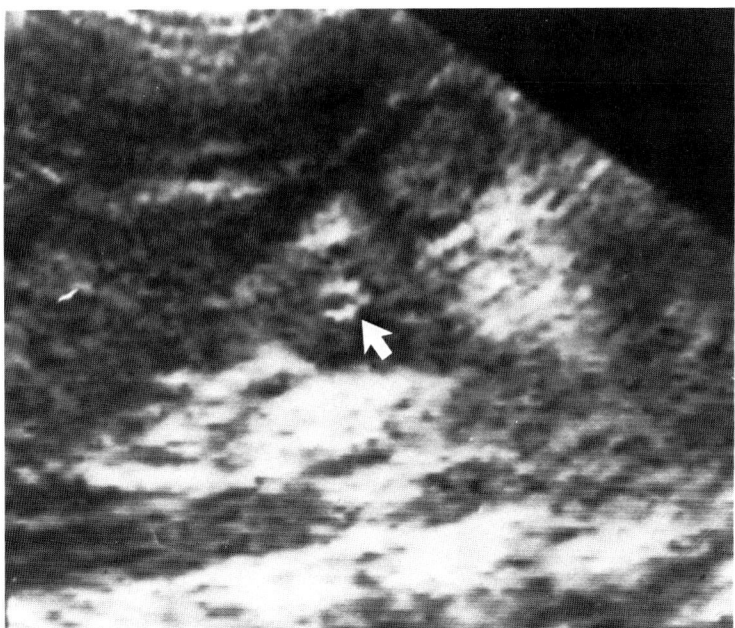

FIGURE 13.2. Longitudinal ultrasonographic images of dilation of the main pancreatic duct (arrow) in a 6-year-old boy with acute pancreatitis (Courtesy of Michael T. Wallach, MD).

reserved for specific recurrent or unusual cases, since uncomplicated acute pancreatitis generally may be expected to resolve and not recur.

CASE PRESENTATION

A 7-year-old previously healthy girl ran hard into a barrier while playing tag at a construction site. No external injuries were sustained and she returned to her play. The next morning she developed severe abdominal pain and vomiting that persisted and increased. On initial examination, she was believed to have a "stomach" virus. No diarrhea occurred. That evening she was brought to an emergency room with continuing symptoms: serum amylase was found to be highly elevated. Ultrasound examination of the abdomen showed dilation of the main pancreatic duct without other abnormalities (Fig. 13.2). She was admitted, placed NPO, and after 3 days peripheral hyperalimentation was begun. Modest doses of pain medication were required for 2 days. The episode of acute pancreatitis resolved without sequelae (Fig. 13.3).

CHRONIC PANCREATITIS

The syndromes of chronic pancreatitis on an idiopathic and familial basis may occur in childhood, as will pancreatitis linked to hyperlipidemia. Children rarely have

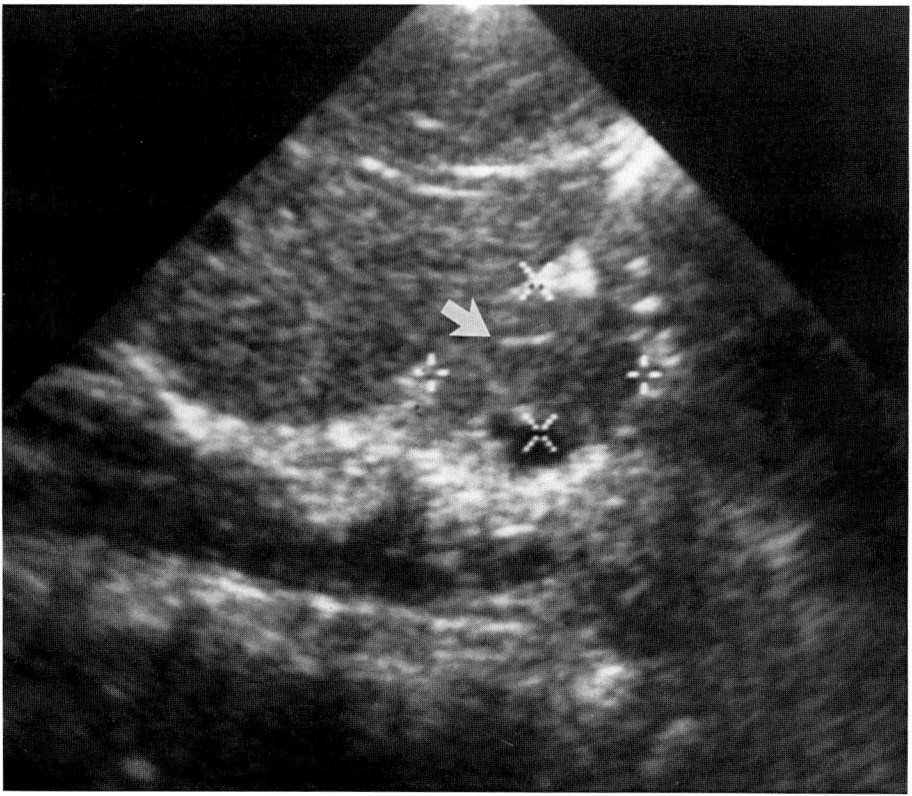

FIGURE 13.3. Same case presented in Figure 13.2 after clinical resolution of acute pancreatitis (Courtesy of Michael T. Wallach, MD).

chronic pancreatitis, and both diagnostic and therapeutic considerations parallel the approach taken in the adult population.

References

1. Silverman R, Roy CC. *Pediatric Clinical Gastroenterology*, 3rd ed. St. Louis: CV Mosby Co., 1983.
2. Lerner A. Hereditary abnormalities of the pancreas. In: Lebenthal E, ed. *Textbook of Gastroenterology and Nutrition in Infancy*, 2nd ed. New York: Raven Press, 1989:877–883.
3. Lloyd-Still JD. Cystic fibrosis. In: Lebenthal E, ed. *Textbook of Gastroenterology and Nutrition in Infancy*, 2nd ed. New York: Raven Press, 1989:831–876.
4. Lemna WK, Feldman GL, Kerem B-S, et al. Mutation analysis for heterozygote detection and the prenatal diagnosis of cystic fibrosis. *N Engl J Med* 1990;322:291–296.
5. Rommens JM, Iannuzzi MC, Kerem B-S, et al. Identification of the cystic fibrosis gene: chromosome walking and jumping. *Science* 1989;245:1059–1065.

6. Riordan JR, Rommens JM, Kerem B-S, et al. Identification of the cystic fibrosis gene: cloning and characterization of complementary DNA. *Science* 1989;245:1066–1073.
7. Kerem B-S, Rommens JM, Buchanan JA, et al. Identification of the cystic fibrosis gene: genetic analysis. *Science* 1989;245:1073–1080.
8. Adelson JW. Pathophysiology of the pancreas in cystic fibrosis. *J Ped Gastroenterol Nutr* 1984;3:574–578.
9. Hadorn B. The exocrine pancreas. In: Anderson CM, Burke V, eds. *Pediatric Gastroenterology*. Oxford: Blackwell Scientific, 1975.
10. Kopelman H, Durie P, Gaskin K, et al. Pancreatic fluid secretion and protein hyperconcentration in cystic fibrosis. *N Engl J Med* 1985;312:329–334.
11. Sokol RJ, Heubi JE, Butler-Simon N, et al. Treatment of vitamin E deficiency during chronic childhood cholestasis with oral d-α-tocopheryl polyethylene glycol-1000 succinate. *Gastroenterology* 1987;93:975–985.
12. Siegel MJ, Martin KW, Worthington JL. Normal and abnormal pancreas in children: U.S. Studies. *Radiology* 1987;165:15–18.

Chapter 14

Carcinoma of the Exocrine Pancreas

RUSSELL YANG
LAURENCE LEICHMAN
PHILIP W. RALLS
HARTLEY COHEN
NARIMAN D. KARANJIA
HOWARD A. REBER

INCIDENCE

Adenocarcinoma of the pancreas often presents with the clinical spectrum of severe pain, cachexia, and depression. Pancreatic cancer is unequalled in the amount of suffering it may cause the patient or the amount of frustration to the physician charged with the care of that patient. In the United States, carcinoma of the pancreas is the fourth leading cause of cancer death in men (after lung, colon, and prostate cancer) and fifth leading cause of cancer death in women (after lung, colon, breast, and uterus/ovary cancer). The mortality of this tumor is high: 86% of patients die within a year of diagnosis and 99% will die of their cancer within 5 years.

The incidence of pancreatic cancer has increased 300% in the last 3 decades in the United States. In Japan, the incidence has risen 4-fold over the same time period. In 1991, it is expected that 28,000 new cases of adenocarcinoma of the pancreas will be discovered in the United States with a slight male predominance (1.7:1).[1] American blacks have a 30% to 40% greater risk of developing this tumor than whites. Similarly, Hawaiian men have double the risk.

Epidemiology

The reasons for the dramatic rise in the incidence of pancreatic cancer are unknown. Epidemiologists have listed cigarette smoking, diabetes mellitus, industrial chemical exposure, alcoholism, diet, radiation exposure, and chronic pancreatitis as putative risk factors for cancer of the pancreas. Of these, cigarette smoking has the strongest and most consistent association with pancreatic carcinoma. Epidemiologic studies demonstrate that men who smoke more than one pack of cigarettes per day have 3 times the risk of developing carcinoma of the pancreas. Similarly, women who smoke more than one pack per day have double the risk for pancreatic cancer. In 50,000 male college students who were followed for up to 50 years, cigarette smoking during their college days was calculated to give a relative risk of 2.6 for developing pancreatic carcinoma.[2] Moreover, workers who have been exposed to asbestos and who smoked developed pancreatic cancer at a higher rate than those workers exposed to asbestos but who did not smoke. Additionally, Weiss and Bernarde studied the temporal pattern of smoking and pancreatic cancer rates.[3] Concomitant changes in pancreatic cancer rates occurred with the rise and fall of cigarette smoking. Thus, epidemiologic studies not only demonstrate an association of cigarette smoking and the development of pancreatic cancer but more importantly, this risk of developing pancreatic cancer appears to be proportional to the quantity of cigarettes smoked.

Further evidence that smoking is associated with the development of pancreatic cancer is provided by autopsy studies. Smokers show histologic alterations in the pancreatic ductal and acinar cells with nuclear atypia as well as advanced hyaline thickening of the arterioles. The severity of these pathologic findings was in direct proportion to the quantity of tobacco smoked. Ductal metaplasia may be the earliest lesion in pancreatic carcinoma.[4]

Pancreatic cancer also appears to be associated with diabetes. Up to 70% of patients with carcinoma of the pancreas manifest glucose intolerance. Most patients with both diabetes and adenocarcinoma of the pancreas exhibited their diabetic condition within 3 months of the diagnosis of their cancer, suggesting that diabetes may constitute an early symptom rather than a predisposing factor. This relationship appears to be more significant in women, although no causal link has yet to be established.[5]

As with breast and large-bowel cancers, several investigators have suggested that diet plays a role in the development of pancreatic carcinoma. Both meat consumption and high-fat diets have been implicated. Interestingly, populations that shun cigarettes, animal fats, and alcohol (ie, Mormons and Seventh Day Adventists) have a lower incidence of pancreatic cancer. Dietary fiber may play a protective role. In addition, MacMahon et al[6] have proposed that drinking coffee regularly is a risk factor for developing pancreatic cancer. The results of this study have not been confirmed by other investigators, and the choice of control patients used in that study (peptic ulcer patients who were told to drink less coffee) may have biased the results. Therefore, coffee ingestion remains to be proven as a strong risk factor for the development of pancreatic cancer.

Industrial exposure to chemicals has been linked to pancreatic carcinoma. Li et al[7] showed that chemists in the United States who worked between 1948 and 1967 had a higher incidence of pancreatic cancer than did age-matched controls. Although Li et al did not document the exact source of exposure, other investigators have associated exposure to solvents (ie, napthylamine and benzidine) and coal tar with an increased incidence of pancreatic carcinoma.[5]

Since up to 4% of patients with carcinoma of the pancreas have pancreatic calcifications, it has been suggested that chronic pancreatitis increases the risk for pancreatic cancer. Except in families with hereditary pancreatitis, where as many as 30% of patients develop pancreatic carcinoma, there is no solid evidence that chronic pancreatitis predisposes a patient to develop pancreatic cancer. Furthermore, no relationship between alcoholism and pancreatic carcinoma has been established.

Genetic factors may also play a role in the development of pancreatic carcinoma. Pancreatic cancer has been reported in familial clusters and in association with other inheritable diseases such as Gardner's syndrome, Lindau's disease, and neurofibromatosis. In the United States blacks and Jews also have a high proportion of pancreatic malignancy.

The mechanism of tobacco-induced pancreatic cancer is not known. Several carcinogens found in tobacco smoke have been identified in experimental animals and include nitrosamines and aromatic hydrocarbons. Wynder et al[8] hypothesize that such carcinogens are absorbed and excreted into the bile by the liver followed by reflux of these agents into the pancreatic duct. Confirmation of such an hypothesis is lacking. In addition, investigators have suggested that cholecystokinin (CCK), a gut hormone that normally stimulates pancreatic growth, may play a role in the genesis of pancreatic carcinoma.

Recently an association between the activation of the *ras* oncogenes and pancreatic carcinoma has been reported.[9] The *ras* gene family is found in several human malignant tumors and encodes a 21 kd protein (p21) that is involved in cell growth and differentiation. Molecular cloning and nucleotide sequencing of the *ras* gene from human tumors have demonstrated that activation of the *ras* oncogene occurs by single point mutations in either codon 12, 13, or 61. Mutations at codon 12 have been associated with the development of pancreatic (90%), colorectal (50%), and lung (25%) adenocarcinomas. These mutations in *ras* can be induced experimentally in animals treated with carcinogens such as methylnitrosurea or dimethylbenz[a]anthracenes. In humans, mutated *ras* oncogenes were observed in 96% of pancreatic carcinomas from autopsy material. Apparently the mutations were found in neoplastic tissue only at both the primary and metastatic sites.[9]

Classification

Although ductal cells are a relatively small component of the pancreas gland, the majority of adenocarcinomas of the pancreatic gland arise from the duct system (Table 14.1). Most pancreatic carcinomas occur in the head of the pancreas (60%), followed by the body (13%) and the tail (5%). They occur in multiple locations in 21% of patients. At the time of diagnosis, most (approximately two thirds) have already developed metastases. Metastases usually occur (in descending frequency) in the liver, lymph nodes, peritoneum, lungs, and pleura.

As noted, almost 90% of primary malignant neoplasms of the nonendocrine pancreas are adenocarcinomas of duct cell origin. Less common cancers that also arise from the duct cells include giant-cell carcinoma, adenosquamous carcinoma, microadenocarcinoma, mucinous (colloid) carcinoma, and cystadenocarcinoma (mucinous). Each has pathologic or clinical features that distinguish it from the prototype duct cell cancer. Malignant tumors of uncertain histogenesis account for about 9% of pancreatic neoplasms. Other malignant lesions arise from the acinar cells (1%) or connective tissue (<1%). A few extremely rare tumors have also been reported (see Table 14.1).

Benign tumors of the pancreas are rare. The most common benign neoplasm of

TABLE 14-1. Primary Malignant Neoplasms of the Nonendocrine Pancreas

Duct Cell Origin	88.8%	Connective Tissue Origin	0.6%
Duct Cell Carcinoma		Leiomyosarcoma	
Giant Cell Carcinoma		Malignant Fibrous	
Adenosquamous Carcinoma		Histiocytoma	
Microadenocarcinoma		Osteogenic Sarcoma	
Mucinous (Colloid)		Fibrosarcoma	
Carcinoma		Rhabdomyosarcoma	
Cystadenocarcinoma		Malignant Neurilemoma	
(Mucinous)		Liposarcoma	
Papillary Cystic Tumor		Uncertain Histogenesis	9.2%
Mucinous–Carcinoid		Pancreaticoblastoma	
Carcinoma		Unclassified	
Carcinoid		Large Cell	
Oncocytic Carcinoid		Small Cell	
Oncocytic Carcinoma		Clear Cell	
Oat-Cell Carcinoma		Malignant Lymphoma	?
Ciliated Cell Carcinoma		Histiocytic	
Acinar Cell Origin	1.2%	Plasmacytoma	
Acinar Cell Carcinoma			
Acinar Cell			
Cystadenocarcinoma			
Mixed Cell Type	0.2%		
Duct–Islet Cell			
Duct–Islet–Acinar Cell			
Acinar–Islet Cell			
Carcinoid–Islet Cell			

Adapted from Cubilla AZ, et al. Cancer of the pancreas (non-endocrine). A suggested morphologic classification. Semin Onc 1979;6:285–297.[10]

the exocrine pancreas is the serous cystadenoma. These are well circumscribed lesions consisting of multiple small cysts ranging in size from microscopic to about 2 cm. Other benign tumors are exceedingly uncommon; a review of the literature reveals only a few examples of each (Table 14.2).[10,11]

Diagnosis

The diagnosis of pancreatic adenocarcinoma is generally not made until the disease is advanced beyond cure. Presenting symptoms include weight loss (90%), pain (75%), jaundice (65%), anorexia (60%), pruritus (40%), and diabetes (15%). Possible physical findings in pancreatic carcinoma are depicted in Figure 14.1. Moosa and Levin[12] have recommended initiation of an evaluation for carcinoma of the pancreas when a patient presents with:

1. Upper abdominal pain and/or back pain consistent with a retroperitoneal origin.
2. Negative gastrointestinal work-up for vague abdominal pain.

TABLE 14.2. **Benign Neoplasms of the Pancreas**

Cystadenoma (Serous, Microcystic)	Hamartoma
Lipoma	Lymphangioma
Fibroma	Perithelioma
Adenoma	Schwannoma
Fibroadenoma	Chromaffinoma
Myoma	Paraganglioma
Myxoma	Neurofibroma
Chondroma	Neurinoma
Hemangioendothelioma	

Adapted from Jordan GL. Benign tumors of the pancreas. In: Howard JM, et al. eds. *Surgical Diseases of the Pancreas.* Philadelphia: Lea & Febiger; 1987.[11]

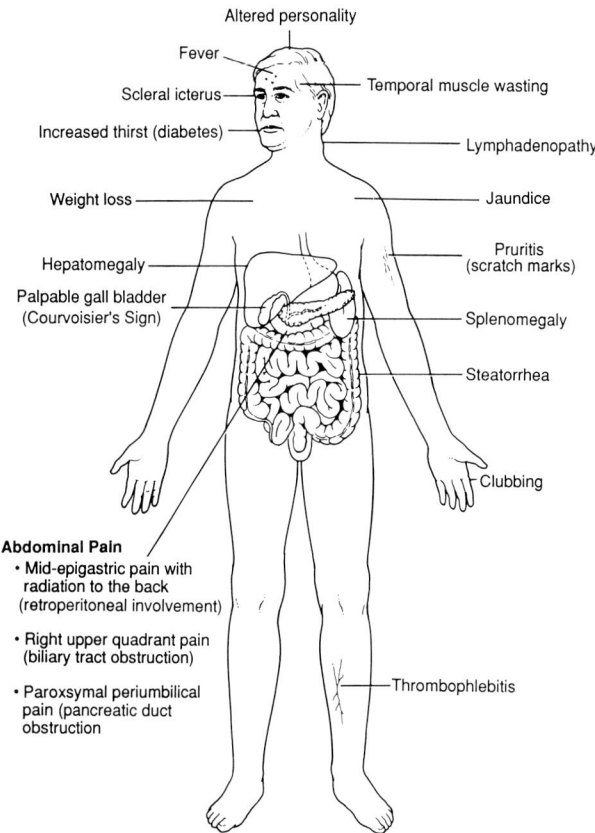

FIGURE 14.1. Possible findings in pancreatic cancer.

3. Obstructive jaundice.
4. Unexplained weight loss of up to 5% of usual body weight.
5. Symptoms of pancreatitis in the absence of gallstone disease or alcohol abuse.
6. New onset diabetes in a patient who is neither obese nor has a family history of diabetes.

Prospective studies using these criteria showed that 50% of patients had pancreatic cancer once the investigations were completed.[12]

Despite the development of many new diagnostic techniques, no single method is sensitive or specific enough for the early diagnosis of pancreatic carcinoma. Pancreatic imaging techniques, pancreatic secretory studies, cytologic examination of duodenal fluid or of pure pancreatic juice, and serum tumor markers have all been employed towards this goal.

Serum Testing

Routine serologic and biochemical tests are nonspecific and cannot reliably diagnose the presence of carcinoma of the pancreas. Alkaline phosphatase, transaminases, and bilirubin are elevated in patients with pancreatic disease but these tests lack the specificity to exclude more benign processes. Therefore, many investigators sought to develop a sensitive and specific marker in serum or pancreatic juice for pancreatic cancer. Potential uses for such a marker include diagnostic screening of high-risk populations or patients with nonspecific signs or symptoms possibly due to pancreatic carcinoma; aiding in the decision of whether to resect the pancreas in patients with a pancreatic mass (particularly if a tissue diagnosis cannot be made before resection); and aiding in evaluation of the efficacy of treatment (ie, the marker would reflect overall tumor burden). Additionally, if high levels correlate with a large tumor burden, then assay of a serum marker may aid in selection of patients with pancreatic cancer who are candidates for surgical exploration.

Markers of pancreatic carcinoma which have been studied include carcinoembryonic antigen (CEA), alpha-fetoprotein (AFP), pancreatic oncofetal antigen (POA), pancreatic RNase, human chorionic gonadotropin (HCG), galactosyltransferase isoenzyme II (GT-II), and CA 19-9.

AFP, POA, HCG, pancreatic ribonuclease, and galactosyl transferase do not appear to be clinically useful in determining the diagnosis or resectability of pancreatic cancer. CEA is a glycoprotein with a molecular weight of 180 kd. Increased levels of CEA arise from rapid tumor growth, an enhanced rate of production, and inability of the liver to clear circulating CEA. In pancreatic cancer, up to 85% of patients have an elevated CEA level; however, high CEA levels are also found in 65% of patients with other neoplasms and in 46% of patients with benign disease such as inflammatory bowel disease, chronic pulmonary disease, and chronic pancreatitis. Nevertheless, high levels of CEA may indicate tumor unresectability. Thus, measurement of CEA levels is not specific or sensitive enough for the screening or diagnosis of pancreatic cancer but may play a role in monitoring the progression of the tumor.

CA 19-9 has been the subject of intense investigation as a tumor marker for carcinoma of the pancreas. CA 19-9 is a monoclonal antibody to a determinant of the Lewis blood group antigen. Elevated levels are found in patients with pancreatic, colorectal, and gastric carcinoma. Overall, CA 19-9 has a specificity of 90% with a sensitivity 80%.[13]

Pancreatic Secretion Testing

Because most human pancreatic carcinomas arise from ductal cells, duodenal aspirates for chemical and cytologic analysis were initially used for the diagnosis of pancreatic malignancy. Duodenal aspirate cytology is only positive in less than 25% of the patients with pancreatic carcinoma. With endoscopic cannulation of the pancreatic duct that yields pure pancreatic juice for cytology, positive results are found in 80% of patients. Better yields are obtained when 3 ml of pancreatic juice were aspirated, when the cannula is inserted deeply in the pancreatic duct, when high suction is applied, when aspiration follows secretin stimulation, and when an intraductal rasp or brush is used. Thus, negative cytologies do not exclude pancreatic carcinomas (low sensitivity) but positive cytologies are strongly suggestive (high specificity).

Changes in pancreatic secretory composition have been investigated. An obstructive pattern with low volume effluent with normal bicarbonate and enzyme output is associated with pancreatic carcinoma. Pancreatic stimulation with secretin and CCK does not distinguish advanced cases of chronic pancreatitis from pancreatic cancer.

IMAGING

Pancreatic imaging has progressed remarkably in the past 15 years with the advent and constant improvement of computed tomography (CT), diagnostic ultrasonography (US), and direct cholangiographic techniques. Initially clinical investigators had hoped that these improvements would allow for early detection of small, curable pancreatic carcinomas; however, it is now clear that modern imaging has had little or no impact on the long-term survival of patients with pancreatic carcinoma. Despite this, imaging (particularly CT) has significantly changed the diagnosis and management of these patients. These advances include improved detection of the initial lesion, confirmation of the diagnosis by guided percutaneous biopsy, assessing its resectability, and following response to therapy.

Lesion Detection

US and CT are the primary tools used to detect pancreatic carcinoma. Although CT is generally the superior imaging modality in these patients, US is useful in certain clinical situations. For example, when a pancreatic head carcinoma causes biliary obstruction, diagnostic US is likely to be the initial imaging test requested and usually succeeds in detecting the obstructing pancreatic carcinoma. In addition, US may also

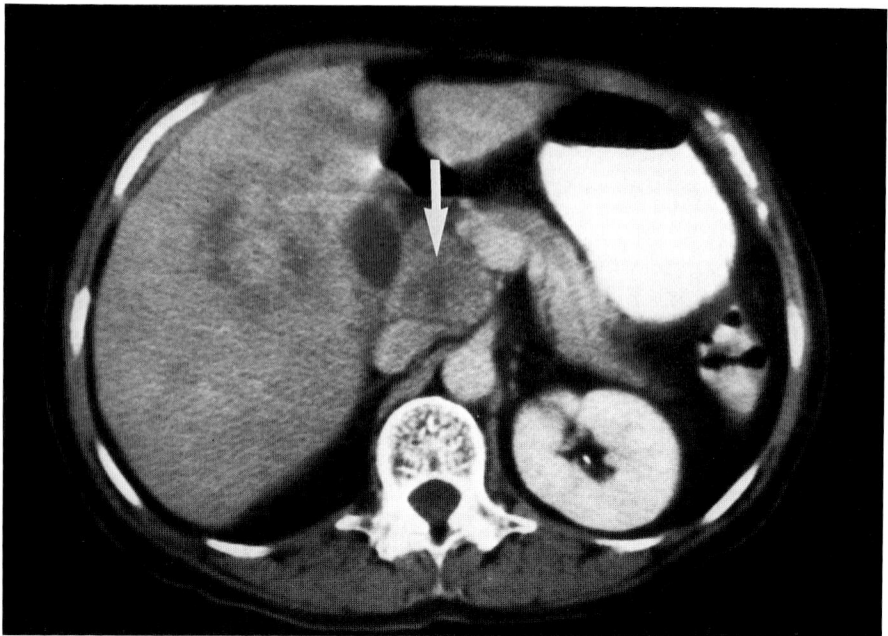

FIGURE 14.2. CT appearance of pancreatic carcinoma. The mass in the head of the pancreas is identified by low density areas (compared with the surrounding enhanced parenchyma) with distortion of gland contour (arrow). Liver metastasis are also seen.

detect carcinoma of the body or tail if it is performed in the evaluation of abdominal pain.

Pancreatic carcinoma appears sonographically as a hypoechoic mass with distortion of the shape of the gland. Other findings include ductal dilation (both common bile and pancreatic ducts), vascular and extraglandular invasion; and metastatic disease. Unlike US imaging of the pancreas, which is frequently limited by overlying bowel gas, CT scanning routinely images the entire pancreas. The hallmark of pancreatic carcinoma on CT is the appearance of a mass. Masses are usually identified by low density areas compared with the surrounding enhanced pancreatic parenchyma, distortion of the architecture of the gland, or both (Fig. 14.2). Pancreatic carcinoma is almost always focal although diffuse lesions have been observed. The lower density areas within the mass are presumably due to fibrosis or necrosis. Additional CT findings of pancreatic adenocarcinoma include dilation of the common bile duct, the pancreatic duct, or both; pancreatic cysts representing pseudocysts (approximately 10%) or cystic necrosis (Fig. 14.3); vascular encasement; extrapancreatic invasion; and metastatic disease (usually to the liver).

False positive diagnosis are possible. Chronic pancreatitis may be seen as a mass effect and ductal dilation (Fig. 14.4). In addition, other pancreatic neoplasms and metastases can occasionally simulate pancreatic adenocarcinoma. Optimal CT sensitivity for pancreatic carcinoma is best achieved using bolus intravenous contrast injection (preferably with a mechanical injector) to accentuate vessel morphology.

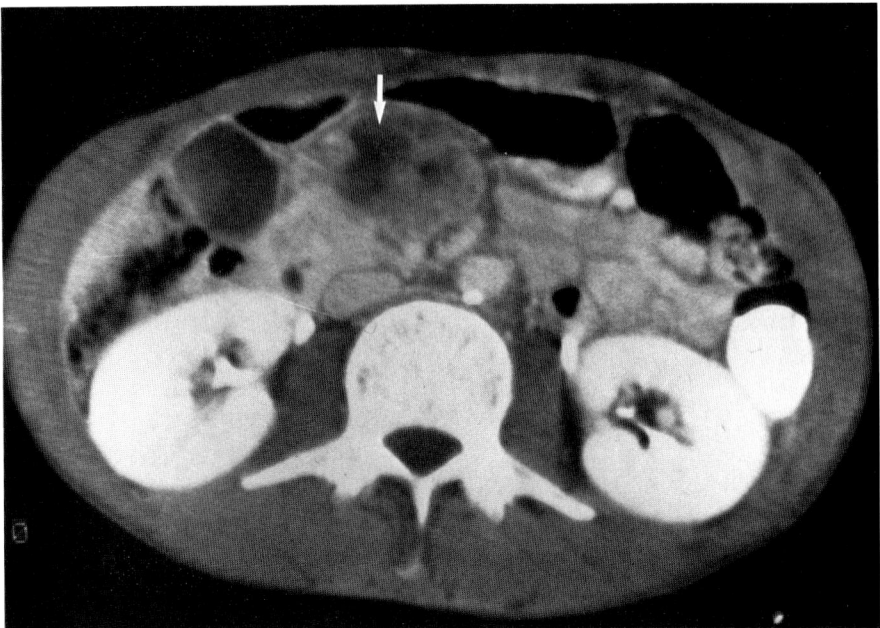

FIGURE 14.3. CT findings of pancreatic adenocarcinoma with cystic necrosis (arrow).

Fine-Needle Aspiration Biopsy

Biopsy is often used to confirm the diagnosis of pancreatic carcinoma and to differentiate it from other masses that occasionally mimic carcinoma. Percutaneous needle aspiration biopsy can be guided successfully by US or CT, and this is a major reason for their diagnostic importance in pancreatic carcinoma.

Determination of Resectability

An important role of CT in patients with pancreatic carcinoma is to assess resectability. Appropriate nonoperative management can be planned in some patients who are determined to be unresectable by CT. The majority of patients believed to be resectable by CT are subsequently found to be unresectable at the time of surgery, however. This is usually because of metastases in normally sized lymph nodes or extrapancreatic invasion were not seen. CT criteria for unresectability includes a lesion that penetrates the capsule and invades surrounding tissue, vascular invasion (obliteration of the fat plane between the tumor and any adjacent vessels, especially the superior mesenteric artery), enlarged lymph nodes (greater than 1.0 cm.), metastases, or evidence of malignant ascites.

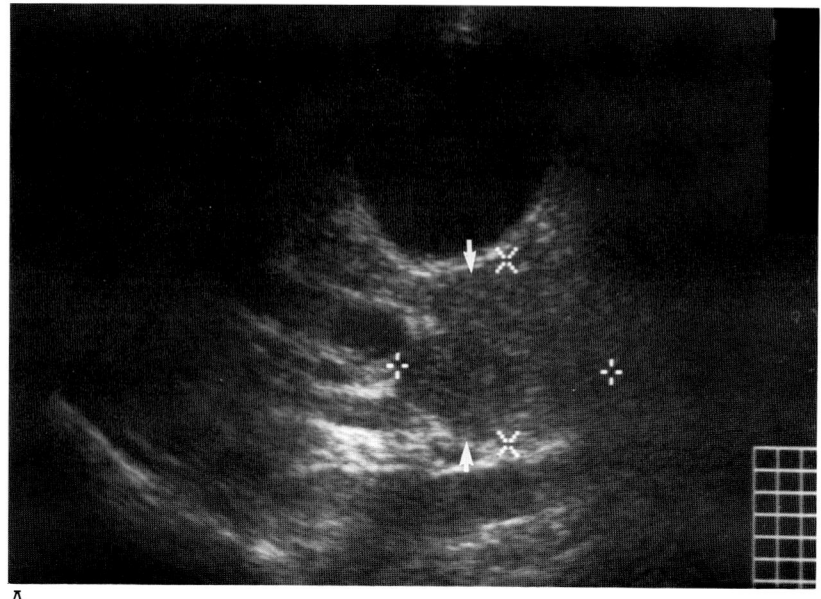

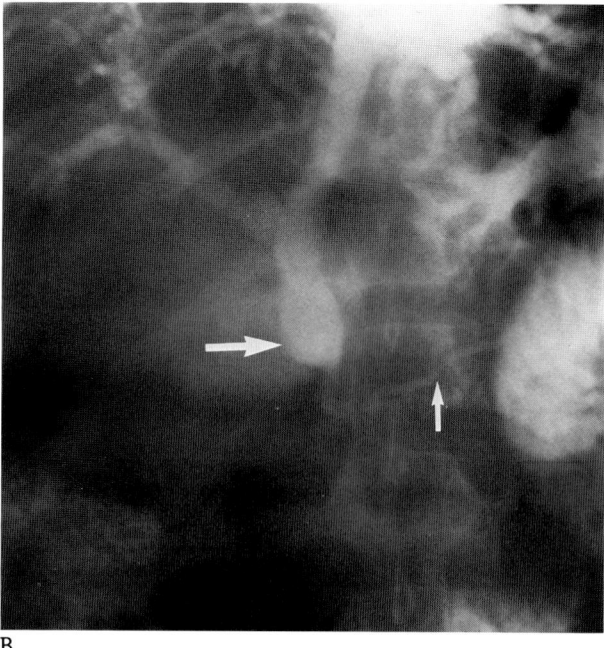

FIGURE 14.4. Pancreatic mass observed in a case of chronic pancreatitis. US (A) demonstrates a mass effect in the head of the pancreas (arrows). No calcifications were seen. Cholangiogram (B) obtained by ERCP demonstrates dilation of the biliary tree (large arrow) and pancreatic duct (small arrow) with obstruction in the distal common bile duct secondary to the pancreatic mass.

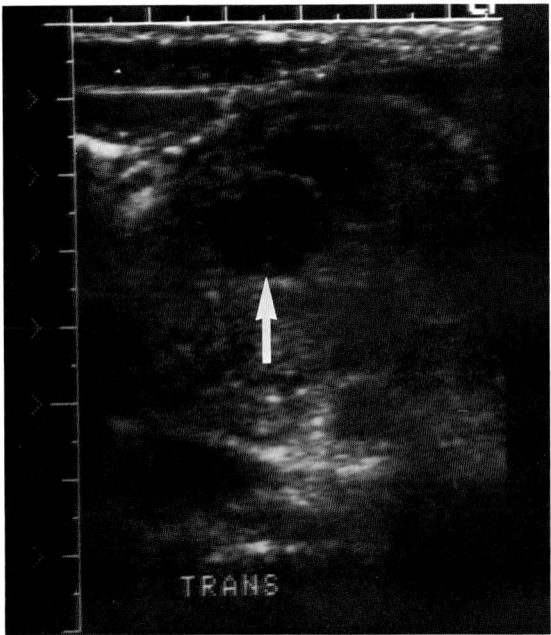

FIGURE 14.5. US findings of a case of pancreatic mucinous cystadenocarcinoma. Internal septations are seen (arrow).

Response to Therapy

Because CT is technically simple and reproducible, it is an effective modality to monitor the response of unresectable pancreatic carcinoma to chemotherapy. Lesion size can be accurately measured on sequential scans. CT is also a useful surveillance tool for following patients who have undergone resection for cure.

Other Neoplasms

Pancreatic ductal adenocarcinomas comprise more than 95% of epithelial pancreatic neoplasms and more than 90% of all pancreatic neoplasms. Many variants of pancreatic ductal adenocarcinoma (adenosquamous carcinoma, anaplastic carcinoma, and pleomorphic giant-cell carcinoma), other rare pancreatic neoplasms, metastases (melanoma, breast, and lung), and lymphoma are sometimes radiographically indistinguishable from ductal adenocarcinoma. Cystic pancreatic neoplasms are the most common tumor that appears differently on imaging. Mucinous cystic tumors are comprised of large cystic masses, usually with internal septations (Fig. 14.5). These tumors may be either benign or malignant. When visualized by CT scanning, serous cystadenomas (microcystic adenoma) are comprised of many small cysts and frequently exhibit a stellate central scar (Fig. 14.6). In about half of these lesions, calcification is seen.

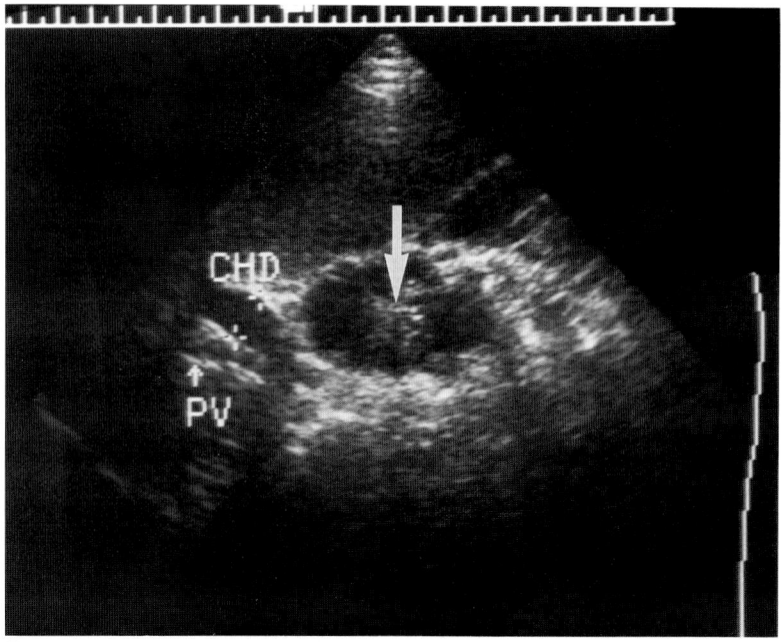

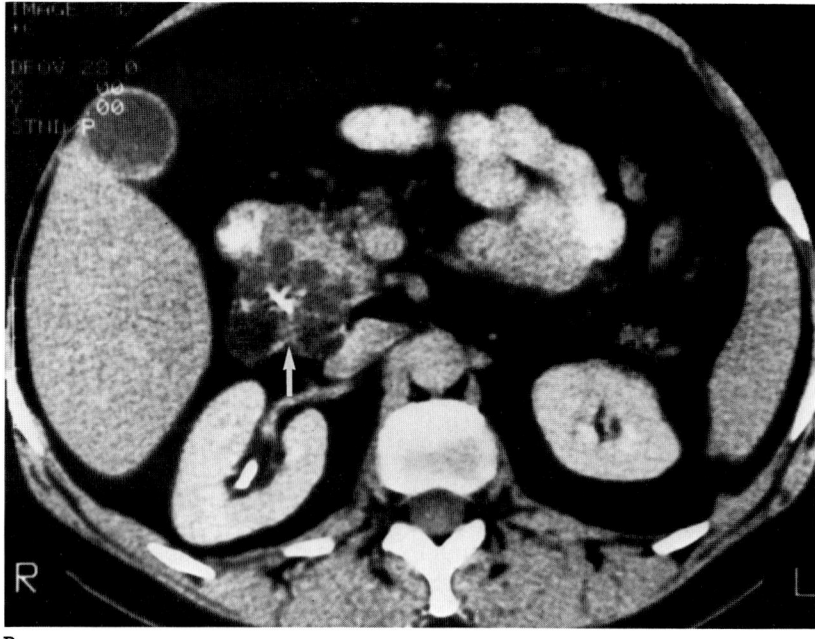

FIGURE 14.6. US (A) and CT (B) appearance of microcystic (serous) cystadenoma of the pancreas. Multiple small cysts and stellate central scar (arrow) are seen. Common hepatic duct (CHD) and portal vein (PV) are labeled on US.

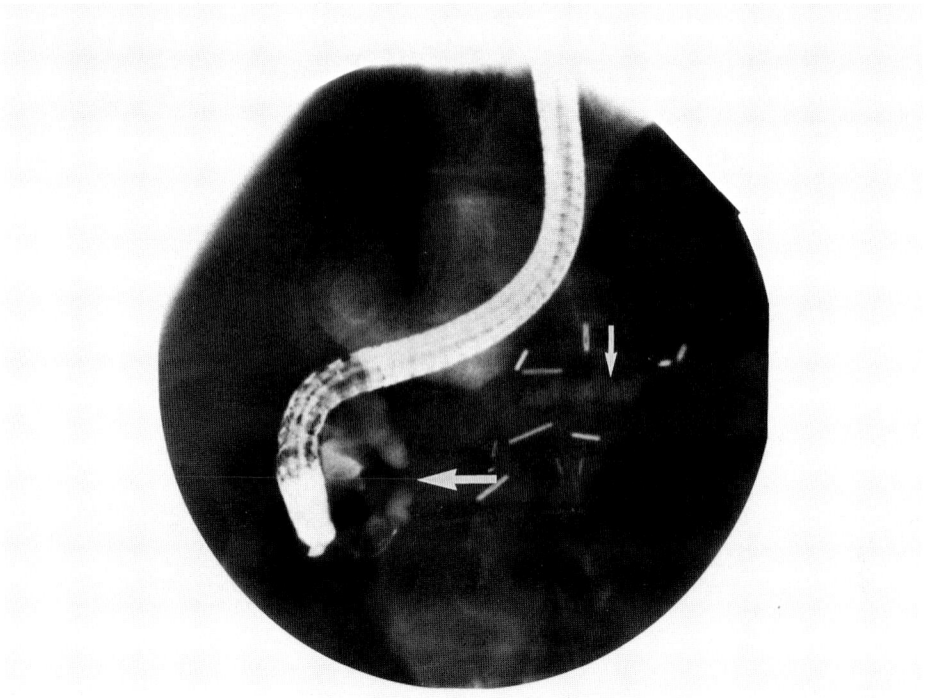

FIGURE 14.7. ERCP showing "double duct" sign of pancreatic carcinoma. Note short stricture of common bile duct (large horizontal arrow) and contrast in dilated distal portion (vertical arrow) of pancreatic duct, which has a long proximal stricture.

Endoscopic Retrograde Cholangiopancreatography

As a diagnostic test for pancreatic carcinoma, endoscopic retrograde cholangiopancreatography (ERCP) is probably more sensitive and specific than either US or CT scanning. In most cases, however, it is not necessary to perform an ERCP since either US or CT studies will detect the presence of a pancreatic mass and allow for image-guided percutaneous pancreatic biopsies (see previous section on imaging). When an ERCP is performed, simultaneous involvement of both pancreatic and bile ducts (ie, the "double duct" sign) is often demonstrated in association with carcinoma of the head of the pancreas (Fig. 14.7).

The major role of ERCP in the management of patients with pancreatic carcinoma is as a therapeutic modality in unresectable disease. Studies demonstrate that endoscopic placement of biliary stents in patients with malignant obstructive jaundice provides satisfactory palliation compared with surgical bypass.

The practice of endoscopic placement of biliary stents has become relatively standardized. Once a tumor has been diagnosed and deemed unresectable an ERCP is performed to image the strictured or obstructed common bile duct. A sphincterotomy is often performed and, using a therapeutic ERCP endoscope (with a biopsy/catheter channel of 4.2 mm), a guide wire is inserted through the common bile duct

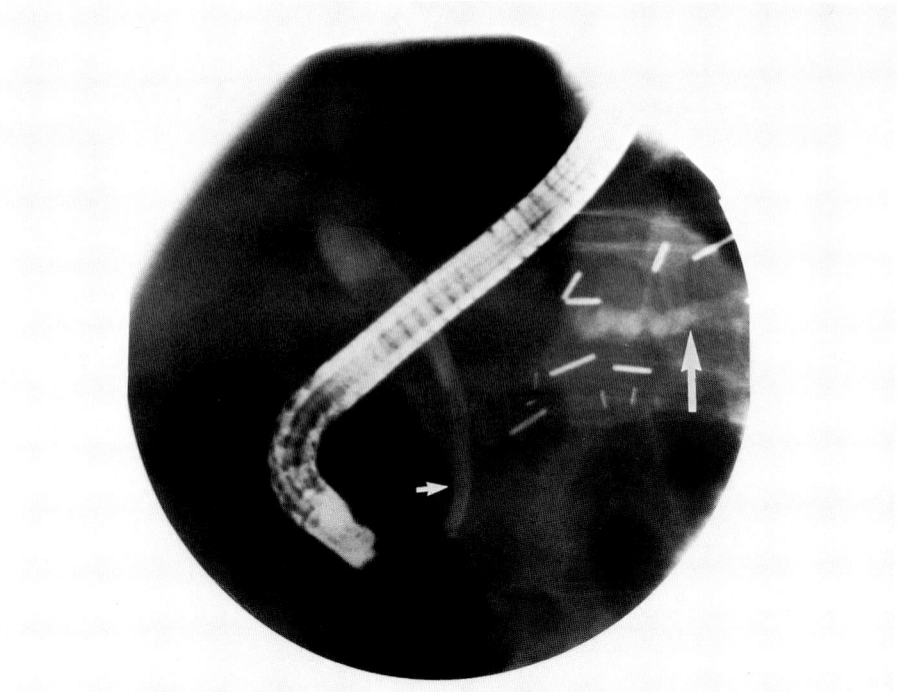

FIGURE 14.8. Same case as Figure 14.7. Note 11.5 Fr stent (horizontal arrow) positioned at common bile duct, traversing stricture shown in Figure 14.7. Residual contrast is present in the dilated distal pancreatic duct (vertical arrow).

stricture. A large-bore stent (10 Fr to 12 Fr) then is pushed over the guide wire through the narrowed common bile duct to allow for adequate biliary drainage into the duodenum (Fig. 14.8). In about 20% of cases, it is not possible to advance the guide wire through the obstruction and a percutaneous transhepatic approach must be used in conjunction with ERCP. In this situation, a guide wire is placed transhepatically down into the duodenum through the narrowing. The duodenoscope is then passed in the usual way into the duodenum and the guide wire is lassoed and pulled through the scope. A stent is then inserted (endoscopically) over the guide wire. The percutaneous part of the technique can be accomplished using a "skinny needle" (20-gauge or smaller) and a 5-Fr catheter with a guide wire. The combined transhepatic–endoscopic technique appears to have some advantage over an exclusively percutaneous technique because it does not involve passage of a large stent through the liver parenchyma and therefore is much less traumatic.

Unfortunately, regardless of which technique is used, currently available stents (even large-bore stents) tend to occlude with debris and bacteria after about 4 months. Thus, routine stent exchanges must be performed every 4 to 6 months, or sooner if the patient has a rising bilirubin or has symptoms or signs of cholangitis. A small number of these patients (approximately 20%) will subsequently require surgery for an enteric bypass surgical drainage (ie, gastrojejunostomy) because of symptomatic duodenal obstruction.

CASE PRESENTATION

A 66-year-old man complained of epigastric pain radiating to the back associated with weight loss of 16 lb. A CT scan of the abdomen was interpreted as suspicious for a mass in the head of the pancreas. The patient underwent an exploratory laparotomy, at which time a midbody pancreatic mass was found with involvement of the superior mesenteric vessels. A biopsy was read as adenocarcinoma and the mass was believed to be unresectable. Three months later the patient became jaundiced. An ERCP was performed (see Fig. 14.7) and a biliary stent was inserted endoscopically (see Fig. 14.8). Jaundice was immediately relieved. The patient died 14 months later. The tumor had involved the duodenal mucosa and persistent bleeding occurred.

AN APPROACH TO THE DIAGNOSIS OF PANCREATIC CARCINOMA

In light of the variety of diagnostic tests and procedures available for the diagnosis of carcinoma of the pancreas, a summary of our approach is diagrammed in Figure 14.9.

Although abdominal US can adequately image the pancreas, it is dependent on the skill of the operator and the body habitus of the patient. US may reveal secondary abnormalities caused by the tumor such as bile duct dilation or a pancreatic mass. Overlying bowel gas often obscures visualization of the pancreas. If abdominal computerized tomography (CT) imaging is inadequate, then an endoscopic retrograde pancreatography (ERP) may be performed. Serum tumor markers and pancreatic secretory tests are optional and do not add to this diagnostic regimen. This approach is successful in more than 90% of patients for distinguishing between pancreatitis and pancreatic cancer.

TREATMENT

The principles of treatment for adenocarcinoma of the pancreas do not differ from those for other common solid tumors and are dictated by the stage of the tumor. Can the patient be cured by surgical intervention? Does surgery offer palliation? Are there other methods for cure, improvement of survival, or palliation? Unfortunately the answers are not always obvious in the setting of pancreatic cancer.

Staging systems are used to guide treatment. The international Tumor Node Metastasis (TNM) Classification adequately prognosticates lesions but is cumbersome

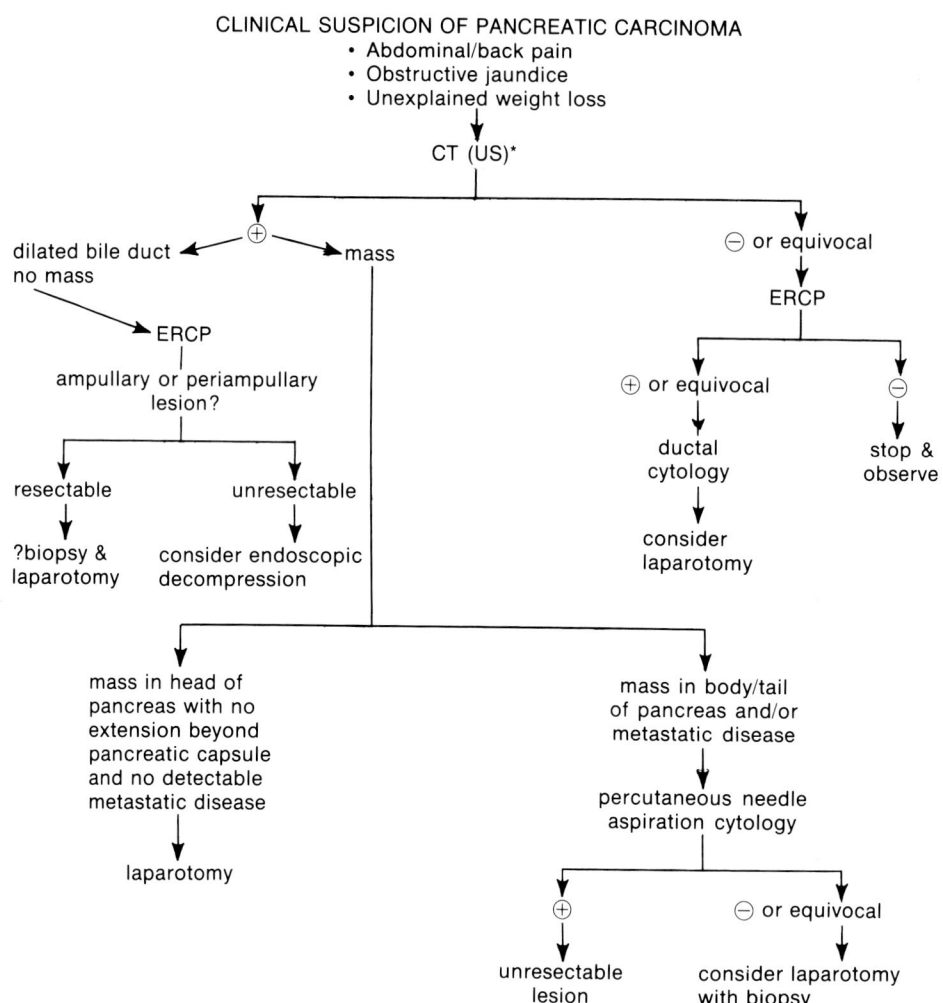

*If performed by an experienced radiologist, US may be as useful as CT in evaluating patients for pancreatic carcinoma. However, adequate US imaging of the pancreas greatly depends on the skill of the operator and on the body habitus of the patient. Overlying bowel gas frequently impairs complete US visualization of the pancreas.

FIGURE 14.9. An approach to the diagnosis and management of pancreatic cancer.

to apply. In the TNM classification system, tumor status is defined by extension through the pancreatic capsule; nodal status is defined by the presence of regional pancreatic lymph involvement; and metastatic status is defined by the presence of distant nodal, peritoneal, or visceral metastases. The classification is as follows:

T1—No direct extension of primary tumor beyond the pancreas
T2—Limited direct extension to duodenum, bile duct, stomach
T3—Advanced direct extension, incompatible with resection

2TX—Direct extension not assessed
N0—Regional lymph nodes not involved
N1—Regional lymph nodes involved
N2—Regional lymph nodes not assessed
M0—No distant metastasis
M1—Distant metastasis present
M2—Distant metastasis not assessed

Because of the awkwardness of this system, many clinicians prefer a simplified classification:

Stage I—Confined to pancreas alone (13-month survival)
Stage II—Involving neighboring structures only (7-month survival)
Stage III—Involving regional lymph nodes (5-month survival)
Stage IV—Including liver or other distant spread (2-month survival)

Surgery for Adenocarcinoma of the Pancreas

In the experience of most pancreatic surgeons, only about 20% of patients with pancreatic cancer have tumors suitable for resection and possible cure at the time of diagnosis.[14]

Carcinoma of the pancreas is considered surgically resectable if the following areas are free of tumor: the hepatic artery near the origin of the gastroduodenal artery; the portal and superior mesenteric veins, and the superior mesenteric artery as they pass behind the pancreas; and the liver or regional lymph nodes. Because of the proximity of the tumor to these structures, their involvement usually occurs early in most cases.

In the majority of cases, a histologic diagnosis is made either preoperatively by percutaneous fine-needle aspiration, or at operation by needle or wedge biopsy or aspiration cytology. This may not be possible, however, particularly with small lesions in the head of the pancreas where a zone of chronic inflammation may surround the tumor. In this situation, decisions about whether to proceed with a resection may have to be made on the basis of indirect evidence for the diagnosis of cancer.

For resectable lesions in the head of the pancreas, the operation of choice is the Whipple pancreaticoduodenectomy (Figs. 14.10.1, .2, .3).[11] This involves the removal of the head of the pancreas (as far as the midbody), the distal stomach and duodenum, the gallbladder, distal common bile duct, and usually a truncal vagotomy (to avoid marginal ulceration). Gastrointestinal continuity is restored with a pancreaticojejunostomy, a choledochojejunostomy, and a gastrojejunostomy. In an effort to minimize the nutritional disturbances of the operation, some surgeons preserve the distal stomach and pylorus, which obviates the need for vagotomy. The benefits of such an approach are unproven, however. Experienced pancreatic surgeons who routinely perform Whipple's procedure have mortality rates less than 5%. Death is usually associated with postoperative complications such as pancreatic and biliary fistulas, hemorrhage, and infection. Overall, the 5-year survival rate for cancer of the head

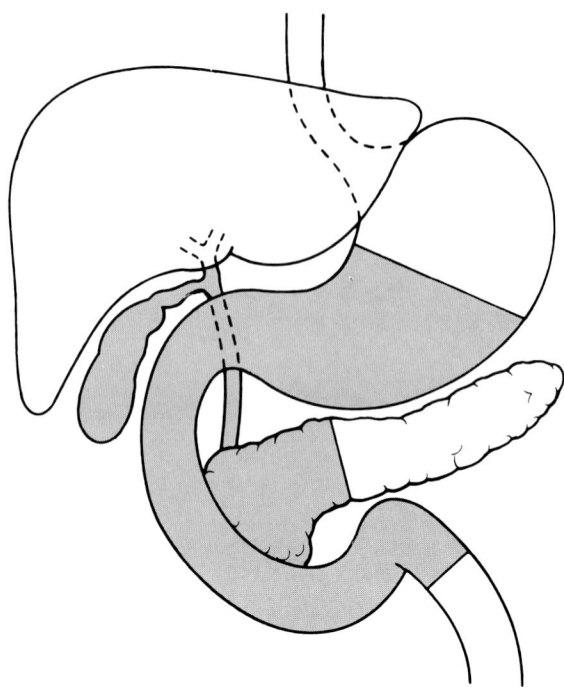

FIGURE 14.10.1. The shaded areas represent the structures that will be removed surgically (distal stomach, duodenum, proximal jejunum, head of pancreas, gall bladder, and common bile duct).

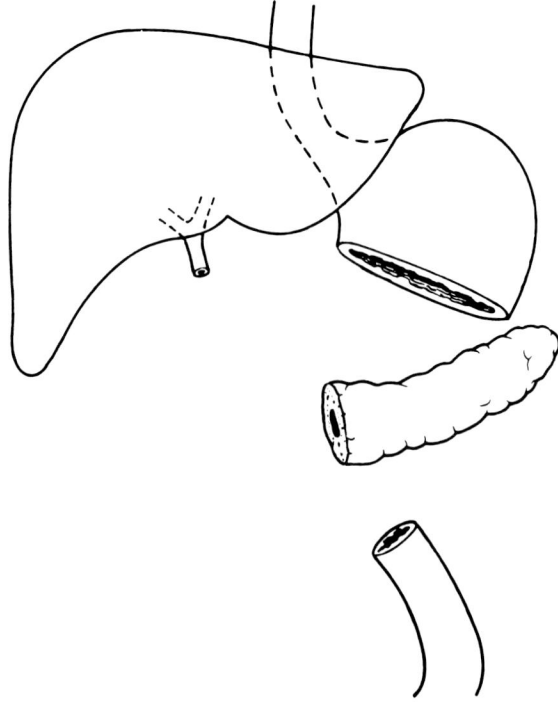

FIGURE 14.10.2. The structures have been removed, and gastrointestinal continuity must be restored.

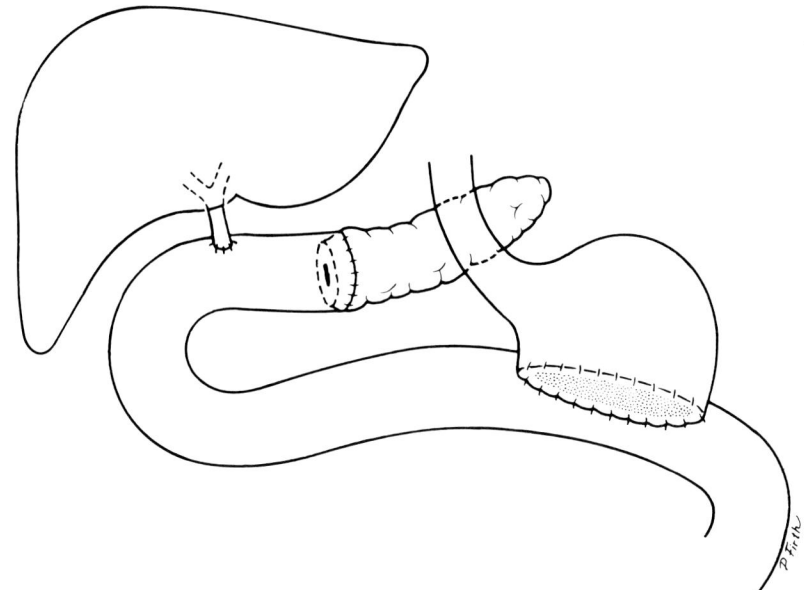

FIGURE 14.10.3. Gastrointestinal continuity is restored with a pancreaticojejunostomy (1), choledochojejunostomy (2), and a gastrojejunostomy (3).

of the pancreas treated with resection is 7% to 10% even though some of these patients are not disease-free.[11] In the case of a lesion in the body or tail of the pancreas, the prognosis is even more dismal.

Palliation

The majority of patients with pancreatic cancer whose lesions are unresectable still require palliation for jaundice, gastric outlet obstruction, or both.

Obstructive jaundice occurs in approximately 70% of all patients with pancreatic cancer at some time during the course of their disease. In patients with carcinoma in the head of the pancreas, jaundice is present in 90% of patients and is due to tumor compression of the common bile duct as it passes through pancreatic tissue. Jaundice is less common in cancers of the body and tail (occurring in less than 6% of such patients). In this situation, jaundice is usually caused by impingement of the common bile duct by involved nodes at the porta hepatis or diminished liver function from liver metastases.

Jaundice should be relieved by either endoscopic (see previous section on ERCP) or surgical drainage for several reasons. First, prolonged jaundice impairs liver function and may result in liver failure. Second, although more common with obstructive jaundice secondary to calculous biliary disease, cholangitis develops in about 10% of patients with unrelieved biliary obstruction caused by malignant disease. Third, malabsorption may ensue leading to anorexia and malnutrition. Fourth, about 25% of jaundiced patients suffer from intractable pruritus that is often impossible to treat effectively with medications alone. Finally, there is presumptive evidence that relief of jaundice may prolong survival. Sarr and Cameron[15] reviewed 10,000 patients who underwent palliative procedures for pancreatic cancer and found that the mean survival time in patients palliated with surgical biliary bypass was 5.4 months compared with 3.5 months in those who did not. It is unclear from this study if patients with more advanced disease were randomized equally between treatment groups, however.

The different internal bypass procedures use either the common bile duct or the gallbladder on the biliary side and the duodenum or jejunum on the intestinal side. External drainage through a surgically placed T-tube provides effective relief of the jaundice but most patients do not prefer living with an external biliary fistula. If large volumes of bilious fluid are lost, severe fluid and electrolyte imbalance can occur. Although this can be corrected by refeeding of bile, most patients find this unacceptable.

Both cholecystoduodenostomy and choledochoduodenostomy have been used to bypass malignant obstructive jaundice. The palliative effectiveness with either procedure is limited because the anastomosis lies too close to the tumor mass and the tumor subsequently spreads to that area. Conversely, choledochoduodenostomy is an effective procedure to bypass biliary obstruction from benign conditions (eg, choledocholithiasis).

Cholecystojejunostomy and choledochojejunostomy are preferred for the relief of obstructive jaundice in patients with periampullary malignancy.[11,16] Both procedures are equally effective and safe, and patients have a mean survival of about 6 months. Before using the gallbladder for decompression, the surgeon must demonstrate patency between the cystic and common bile ducts. If the tumor has obstructed this area, the gallbladder should not be used and the common duct can be selected.

The decision to provide relief of obstructive jaundice by percutaneous or endoscopically placed biliary stents versus surgical drainage should be individualized since all methods provide effective palliation.[17] Stent placement is usually preferred in patients in whom laparotomy may be contraindicated (eg, unacceptable surgical risk, patient refusal, proven unresectable disease). If duodenal obstruction occurs, operative intervention is necessary to relieve it and surgical biliary bypass should be done at that time as well.

Only about 5% to 10% of patients with pancreatic cancer present with duodenal obstruction at the time of diagnosis; an additional 20% of patients will develop duodenal obstruction at some stage of their disease. Duodenal compression or distortion by the tumor can be documented by gastrointestinal endoscopy or roentgenography. In such patients, the need for a gastrojejunostomy is clear. When duodenal obstruction is not present and when operative inspection does not suggest that it may develop soon, however, the value of prophylactic gastrojejunostomy is less clear. In a review of 1000 patients who underwent biliary bypass alone, an average of 21% required reoperation because duodenal obstruction developed 1 to 12 months later.[15,16] Concern that the addition of a gastrojejunostomy to a biliary bypass procedure would increase the operative mortality and morbidity is unjustified. In a collected series of 452 patients undergoing biliary bypass alone, the mortality rate was 17.7% and the mean survival was 6.3 months.[16] In another review of 193 patients who underwent both a biliary bypass and a gastrojejunostomy, the mortality rate was 16.4% and the mean survival was 6.1 months.[16] Thus, most surgeons agree that prophylactic gastrojejunostomy is safe and should be performed in any patient who is likely to survive for at least a few months.

If the patient with pancreatic cancer has significant pain, then a procedure for pain relief may be done at the time of laparotomy. Individual sectioning of the greater and lesser splanchnic nerves; a celiac and superior mesenteric ganglionectomy; or division of the postganglionic celiac plexus from T-5 to T-10 have been tried. Although the early results of each of these procedures have been encouraging, pain relief is often transient. The chemical destruction of the celiac ganglia at operation with 50% ethanol or 6% phenol is simpler and may be more effective. Furthermore, if injection is not effective or only provides transient relief, percutaneous injections of similar agents may be attempted at a later date.

Surgery for Uncommon Tumors of the Pancreas

No clinical or laboratory features allow a preoperative differentiation between uncommon tumors and adenocarcinoma of the pancreas. Certain characteristics should raise the index of suspicion, however. For instance, sarcomas are relatively more frequent in young people and tend to grow considerably larger than duct carcinomas. Giant cell carcinomas, microadenocarcinomas, and cystadenocarcinomas on average are 2 to 3 times the size of the typical ductal cancer. Obstruction of the bile duct and duodenum is less common because many of these lesions arise in the body or tail of the pancreas. These distal lesions often attain significant size without invading adjacent structures. In general, the presence of an unusual pancreatic tumor may be suspected when the tumor is especially large and the patient has not suffered significant weight loss or pain; when percutaneous needle aspiration demonstrates cells atypical of ductal adenocarcinoma; when the patient is less than 40 years of age; when the mass is cystic, especially when it is multilocular or calcified, and the patient has no previous history of chronic pancreatitis; or when angiography demonstrates hypervascularity (typical of cystadenoma and cystadenocarcinoma).

Unlike the usual ductal adenocarcinoma, uncommon tumors of the pancreas may become large without invading adjacent vital structures. In some cases, curative resection of all or part of the pancreas along with adherent organs (eg, colon, stomach) have been reported,[11] suggesting that an aggressive surgical approach is justified. If resection is not advisable, prophylactic biliary bypass and gastrojejunostomy should probably be done because obstruction may occur as the tumor grows. All unresectable tumors should be marked with metal clips to direct postoperative radiotherapy. During the resection of neoplastic cysts, effort should be made to remove the tumor intact since rupture may disseminate cells.

If back pain is present in patients with unresectable tumors, celiac plexus block can be performed. In many cases the size of the tumor or the extent of retroperitoneal involvement precludes successful operative block. In these cases a procedure can be done later through the percutaneous route.[16]

Radiation and Chemotherapy for Adenocarcinoma of the Pancreas

Nonsurgical treatment of unresectable pancreatic carcinoma relies on the combination of radiation and chemotherapy. Patients with localized, unresectable cancer in particular (as many as 40% of patients with pancreatic adenocarcinoma) present the greatest therapeutic challenge since they represent a potentially curable group because they have no known distant metastasis.

Radiation may be administered by external beam, by implantation of radiation seeds, or by fast neutron irradiation. The target volume of external beam radiation includes the primary tumor site and the adjacent 3 to 5 cm of pancreatic tissue, the draining lymph nodes, and for tumors of the pancreatic head, the duodenum. Radiation fields encompass the pancreaticoduodenal, celiac, suprapancreatic, and porta hepatis areas. For lesions of the pancreatic body and tail, the splenic hilum node is included in the field. Field borders are defined by CT scans taken with oral contrast material, by surgical clips placed at laparotomy to mark tumor margins, from descriptions provided in the operative and pathology reports, and when available, by angiographic and ERCP films. The radiation is generally administered in fractionated intervals up to a total dose of 5000 rads. Further radiation may be given to a smaller volume encompassing the gross disease only. Using this approach, Haslam et al[18] obtained a median survival of all treated patients of 7.5 months. Thirty-one percent of patients were alive 18 months after diagnosis, and six patients survived 2.5 years. This suggests that radiation offers more than simple palliation from pain.

Interstitial implantation of radiation seeds has also been used in the palliation of pancreatic carcinoma. For small tumors which can be adequately implanted, total doses of 15,000 rads can be delivered locally, followed by 4000 to 5000 rads of external irradiation. Despite local regional control by this method, however, prolonged survival in these patients has not been demonstrated.

Fast neutron irradiation, a form of high linear energy transfer radiation, has a 3-fold increase on the "radiation effect" on normal and malignant cells compared with routine external beam radiation. The use of this energy source is believed to overcome hypoxic resistance of malignant cells to radiation treatment. Clinical trials are now underway to evaluate its therapeutic efficacy.

Acute complications of upper abdominal radiation therapy are common during treatment and include nausea, vomiting, anorexia, diarrhea, and fatigue. These usually resolve 1 to 2 weeks after therapy is completed. Chronic complications such as gastritis, upper gastrointestinal bleeding, small bowel obstruction, fistula formation, cholangitis, necrotizing pancreatitis, pancreatic insufficiency, diabetes mellitus, and retroperitoneal fibrosis are often difficult to distinguish from progression of the underlying pancreatic carcinoma.

Even when radiation is effective for localized cancer, failure outside the radiation field is the rule. Fifty percent of patients already have cancer outside fields of surgery or radiation when they are initially diagnosed. Thus, the need for effective systemic therapy for pancreatic carcinoma is obvious. The testing of individual chemotherapeutic agents has shown that four classes of agents have marginal, but definitive activity against disseminated pancreatic carcinoma. The antimetabolite 5-fluorouracil (5-FU) has been the most widely tested compound. Overall, 5-FU results in a meaningful response rate of 25%. The therapeutic efficacy of 5-FU has been enhanced by the concomitant administration of compounds such as leucovorin, N-phospho-n-acetyl-L-aspartic acid (PALA), thymidine, allopurinol, or methotrexate. It is common practice to combine 5-FU administration with radiation therapy for cancer of the pancreas since 5-FU is believed to "sensitize" malignant cells to the effects of radiation.[19] Combination therapy can result in a median survival as long as 2 years.

The antibiotic mitomycin-C is also an active agent against pancreatic carcinoma. Single agent response rates for mitomycin are about 25%. Although this agent may be used in jaundiced patients, renal failure precludes its use since mitomycin-C is extensively metabolized by the kidney. Because of its prolonged suppressive effect on the bone marrow, it is difficult to use mitomycin-C in combination with radiation therapy or other agents that may cause similar bone marrow toxicity.

The chlorethylnitrosureas (Carmustine (BCNU), Comustine (CCNU), methyl-CCNU, and streptozotocin) have been tested against disseminated pancreatic cancer with only modest single agent activity. Streptozotocin acts specifically as a pancreatic islet cell toxin and is useful in the treatment of islet cell tumors, with response rates of 31% to 50%.

Adriamycin is an alternative chemotherapeutic agent with an overall response rate of 13%. As with 5-FU, mitomycin-C, and the nitrosureas, responses to adriamycin are brief and usually last less than 12 weeks. Since adriamycin is extracted in the bile, this agent cannot be used in patients with significant biliary obstruction.

In summary, neither radiation nor systemic cytotoxic therapy alone will reliably decrease tumor burden and relieve symptoms for patients with disseminated adenocarcinoma of the pancreas. Combined therapy with these two modalities is more efficacious, however, and can result in an improved quality of life. Absolute proof of prolonged survival is lacking and randomized clinical trials to test the newer treatment modalities are needed. Combination therapy is most beneficial when used adjunctively after tumor resection or in patients with unresectable but localized disease.

References

1. Silverberg E, Boring CC, Squires TS. Cancer statistics, 1990. *CA* 1990;40:9–26.
2. Whittemore AS, Paffenbarger RS, Anderson K, et al. Early precursors of pancreatic cancer in college men. *J Chronic Dis* 1983;36:251–256.
3. Weiss W, Bernarde MA. The temporal relation between cigarette smoking and pancreatic cancer. *Am J Pub Health* 1983;73:1403–1404.
4. Auerbach O, Garfinkel L. Histological changes in pancreas in relation to smoking and coffee drinking habits. *Dig Dis Sci* 1986;31:1014–1020.
5. Boyle P, Hsieh C-C, Maisonneuve P, et al. Epidemiology of pancreas cancer (1988). *Int J Pancreatol* 1989;5:327–346.
6. MacMahon B, Yen S, Trichopoulos D, et al. Coffee and cancer of the pancreas. *New Engl J Med* 1981;304:630–633.
7. Li FP, Fraumeni JF, Mantel N. Cancer mortality among chemists. *J Nat Cancer Inst* 1969;43:1159–1164.
8. Wynder EL, Mabudi K, Maruchi N, et al. A case control study of cancer of the pancreas. *Cancer* 1973;31:641–648.
9. Almoquera C, Shibata D, Forrester K, et al. Most human carcinomas of the exocrine pancreas contain mutant c-K-ras genes. *Cell* 1988;53:549–554.
10. Cubilla AZ, Fitzgerald PJ. Cancer of the pancreas (non-endocrine). A suggested morphologic classification. *Semin Onc* 1979;6:285–297.
11. Jordan GL. Benign tumors of the pancreas. In: Howard JM, Jordan GL, Reber HA, eds. *Surgical Diseases of the Pancreas*. Philadelphia: Lea & Febiger, 1987.

12. Moosa AR, Levin B. The diagnosis of "early" pancreatic cancer—the University of Chicago experience. *Cancer* 1981;47(suppl):1688–1697.
13. Steinberg W. The clinical utility of the CA 19-9 tumor-associated antigen. *Am J Gastroenterol* 1990;85:350–355.
14. Singh SM, Longmire WP Jr, Reber HA. Surgical palliation of pancreatic cancer: the UCLA experience. *Ann Surg* 1990;212:132–139.
15. Sarr MG, Cameron JL. Palliation of pancreatic cancer. *World J Surg* 1984;8:906.
16. Reber HA. Palliative operations for pancreatic cancer. In: Howard JM, Jordan GL Jr, Reber HA, eds. *Surgical Diseases of the Pancreas.* Philadelphia: Lea & Febriger, 1987.
17. Cotton PB. Nonsurgical palliation of jaundice in pancreatic cancer. In: Reber HA, ed. 1989:613–637.
18. Haslam J, Cavanaugh P, Stroup S. Radiation therapy in the treatment of unresectable adenocarcinoma of the pancreas. *Cancer* 1973;32:1342–1345.
19. Gastrointestinal Tumor Study Group. Treatment of locally unresectable carcinoma of the pancreas: comparison of combined-modality therapy (chemotherapy plus radiotherapy to chemotherapy alone). *J Nat Cancer Inst* 1988;80:751–755.

Index

A
Abdominal pain
  in acute pancreatitis, 47
  in chronic pancreatitis, 100–101
  treatment of, 131–133
Abscess, 73–75
  acute pancreatitis and, 26
  preventing, 68
Acetate, 36
Acetylcholine, 70
Acid, 136
Acidosis, 93–94
Acinar cells, 5–10, 16
  acute pancreatitis and, 26–27
  alcohol and, 35
  CCK and, 17
  chronic pancreatitis and, 24
  inhibition of, 69–70
Acute pancreatitis, 23–24
  chronic pancreatitis and, 102–103
  complications of, 87–97
  diagnosis of, 49–54
  management of, 67–72
  pathology of, 25–27
  pseudocyst and, 75
Adenocarcinoma, see Cancer
Adrenergic nerves, 16
Adriamycin, 177
Afferent loop syndrome, 44
Alanine transaminase, 5
Albumin, 87
Alcohol dehydrogenase (ADH), 35
Alcoholic ketoacidosis, 93–94
Alcoholic ketosis, 96
Alcoholic pancreatitis, 5, 34–36, 107–108
Alcoholism, 24, 33, 99, 107
  cancer and, 157
  hyperlipidemia and, 41–42
  treatment and, 131–132
  withdrawal from, 94
Alkaline phosphatase, 5
Alpha amylase, 4
Ampullary carcinoma, 37
Amylase, 1
  diagnosis and, 49–50
  secretion of, 16

Amylolytic enzymes, 4
Analgesia, 133–134
  acute pancreatitis and, 67
Anesthetics, 71
Aneurysms, 106
Anionic trypsinogen, 2
Annular pancreas, 143–145
Antacids, 136
Antibiotics, 68, 74, 76
Anticholinergics, 70, 133
Antrectomy, 14
Aprotinin, 71
Asbestos, 156
Ascites, 106
Aspiration, 62–65, 133
  cancer and, 163
Atrophy, 125–127, 135
Atropine, 13–15, 70
Autophagy, 4
Azathioprine, 39

B
Basal secretion, 11
Basilar atelectasis, 88
Basolateral escape, 32
Basolateral membrane, 7–8
Bicarbonate, 1
  alcohol and, 36
  ductal cells and, 10–11
  inhibition of, 19
  measurement of, 114
  secretion of, 12
Bile
  feedback and, 20–21
  secretion of, 12
Bile ducts
  dilation of, 125
  ERCP and, 167–168
Bile salts, 3
Biliary bypass, 175
Biliary obstruction, 104
Biliary pancreatitis, 56–57
Biliary tract disease, 33–34
Bleeding, see Hemorrhage
Bombesin, 17
Bone marrow, 94

INDEX

C

Calcifications, 43, 99, 125–127
  cancer and, 156
Calcified pancreatitis, 110
Calcitonin gene-related peptide, 19
Calcium, 4, 11, 91–93
Calcium pathway, 7–8
Calculi, 36
Camostate (FOY-305), 71
cAMP, see Cyclic adenosine monophosphate (cAMP) pathway
Cancer, 5, 37, 155–177
  chronic pancreatitis and, 122
  treatment of, 169–177
Carbohydrates, 4
Carboxyl-ester hydrolase, 1
Carboxyl-ester lipase, 3–4
Carboxypeptidase, 1–3
Carcinoembryogenic antigen (CEA), 5, 116
Cardiovascular complications, 87–88
Cassava root, 43, 108–109
Catecholamines, 19
Cationic trypsinogen, 2
CCK, see Cholecystokinin
CEA, see Carcinoembryogenic antigen
Celiac plexus block, 175
Central nervous system, 14, 31
Centroacinar cells, 5, 10–11
Cephalic phase, 13–14
Chemicals, industrial, 156
Chemotherapy, 165, 175–177
Children, 150–152
Chlorethylnitrosureas, 177
Chloride, 1, 145–146
  ductal cells and, 10–11
Chlorothiazide, 39
Cholangitis, 104, 173
Cholecystokinin (CCK), 4–5, 16–18, 32, 114
  blockers, 70
  feedback and, 20–21
  treatment and, 133–134
Choledochocele, 38
Choledochojejunostomy, 171
Cholelithiasis, 23, 150
Cholesterol lipase, 3–4
Cholestyramine, 20
Cholinergic duodenopancreatic reflex, 15
Cholinergic gastro-pancreatic vagovagal reflex, 14
Chronic pancreatitis, 24, 99–110
  in children, 152
  diagnosis of, 113–122
  forms of, 107–110
  pseudocyst and, 75
  treatment of, 131–141
Chyme, 15
Chymotrypsinogen, 1–2
  fecal, 120

Cimetidine, 69, 136
Clinical findings
  of abscess, 73–74
  of acute pancreatitis, 47–58
  in children, 150–151
  of chronic pancreatitis, 100–102
  of injury, 84
  of pseudocyst, 75–76
Coagulation abnormalities, 90–91
Codeine, 134
Coffee, 156
Colipase, 1, 3
Colloids, 87
Colonic phase, 19
Computed tomography (CT), 61–65
  abscess and, 74
  cancer and, 161–165
  chronic pancreatitis and, 125–128
  injury and, 84
  pseudocyst and, 76
Congenital aberrations, 143–145
Congenital pancreatic aplasia, 144
Contrast studies, 61
C-reactive protein (CRP), 54
Creatinine, 96
Crynophagia, 4, 32
Crystalloid solutions, 87
CT, see Computed tomography
Cyanide, 109
Cyclic adenosine monophosphate (cAMP) pathway, 7–9
Cystgastrostomy, 77
Cystic fibrosis, 145–150
Cysts, 24
  bile duct, 38
Cytoplasm, 31–32
Cytoplasmatic extragranular route, 10

D

Denervation, 134–135
Deoxyribonucleases, 3
Diabetes, 24, 101–102
  cancer and, 156
  management of, 137
Diabetic ketoacidosis, 51, 93, 96
Diet, 133
  cancer and, 156
Direct metabolic effect, 35
Distal pancreatectomy, 95%, 141
Diuretics, 39, 82
DNA hybridization method, 146
Down's syndrome, 144
Drug-induced pancreatitis, 38–40
Dual-labeled Schilling test, 118
Ductal system, 10–11, 109
  cancer and, 157

INDEX

dilation of, 125, 132
obstruction of, 36–37
Duodenal aspirate cytology, 161
Duodenal atresia, 143–144
Duodenal diverticula, 37
Duodenal intubation, 114–115
Duodenal obstruction, 174
Duodenopancreatic reflux, 32–33

E

Echogenicity, 61–62
Edematous pancreatitis, 23–24
Effectors, 7
Elastase, 1, 3, 52
Elastin, 3
Electrolytes, 7, 11
  disturbances of, 67–68
Emphysema, 3
Encephalopathy, 94–97
Endocrine insufficiency, 24
Endopeptidases, 2
Endoscopic cannulation, 115–116, 161
Endoscopic drainage, 78, 132, 173
Endoscopic retrograde cholangiopancreatography (ERCP), 41
  acute pancreatitis and, 56–57
  cancer and, 167–169
  chronic pancreatitis and, 122, 127–129
  pseudocyst and, 76
  trauma and, 84
Endoscopic retrograde pancreatography (ERP), 33, 132
Enterokinase, 32
Enzymes, 1–5
  administering, 133–134
  biosynthesis of, 9–10
  cystic fibrosis and, 147
  determination of, 119–120
  diagnosis and, 52
  inactivation of, 70–72
  inhibition of, 19
  measurement of, 114
  secretion of, 5–15
Epidemiology
  of cancer, 155–157
  of chronic pancreatitis, 99
ERCP, see Endoscopic retrograde cholangiopancreatography
ERP, see Endoscopic retrograde pancreatography
Esophagus, 13
Estrogens, 39
Excision, 78
Exocrine insufficiency, 24
Exocytosis-vectorial transport hypothesis, 9–10
Exogenous glucagon, 18–19
Exopeptidases, 2

External drainage, 78, 174
  of abscess, 74
  of ascites, 82

F

Fat necrosis, 25–26, 94
Fatty acids, 4, 42
  deficiency of, 101
  oxidation of, 35
  test with, 118–119
Feedback regulation, 19–21
Fistula, 84
Fluids
  cystic fibrosis and, 146
  leakage of, 81–83
Fluorescein, 117–118
5-Fluorouracil (5-FU), 69, 176
Focal enlargement, 125–127
Function tests, 113–122, 127–128
Furosemide, 39

G

Gabexate mesilate (FOY), 71
Gallbladder, 174
Gallstones, 33–34, 37
  sonography and, 61
Gamma glutamyl transferase, 5
Gardner's syndrome, 157
Gastrectomy, 14
Gastric acid secretion, 12
Gastric phase, 14
Gastrin releasing peptide, 17
Gastrojejunostomy, 171, 175
Glucagon, 70
Glucose, 35

H

Hematemesis, 106
Hemolysis, 31
Hemorrhage, 29, 91
  gastrointestinal, 104–106
  pseudocyst and, 76
  splenic vein, 105–106
Hemorrhagic pancreatitis, 24
  abscess and, 73
Hepatic failure, 44, 104
Hereditary pancreatitis, 43, 110
  cancer and, 156
Heterotopic pancreatic tissue, 144
Histamine, 29
Hormones, 7
  mechanisms of, 16–19
  plasma profile of, 120
Hydrochlorothiazide, 39
Hydrogen breath test, 119
Hydromorphone, 134
Hydroxyzine HCL, 67

INDEX

Hyperamylasemia, 42, 49
Hyperglycemia, 93
Hyperlipasemia, 50–51
Hyperlipidemia, 41–42
Hyperparathyroidism, 42
Hyperphagia, 135
Hypertension, 68, 105
Hypertriglyceridemia, 29, 41–42, 49
Hyperuricosuria, 135
Hypocalcemia, 54, 68, 91–93
Hypoglycemia, 93
Hypokalemia, 93
Hypomagnesemia, 68, 93
Hypoplasia, 144
Hypotension, 54, 87
Hypovolemia, 38, 68, 87
Hypoxemia, 54, 68, 88

I

Idiopathic chronic pancreatitis, 110
Immunoglobulin A (IgA), 5
Increased pancreatic duct permeability hypothesis, 36
Infants, 143–150
Infected phlegmon, see Abscess
Infections, 40, 150
Inflammatory bowel disease (IBD), 52
Ingestion, 11–15
  treatment and, 131–132
Inhibitors, 18–19
Injury, 83–85
Insecticide intoxication, 43–44
Insulin, 3, 18, 93, 96–97
Interdigestive secretion, 11–12
Internal drainage, 78
Intestinal phase, 15
Intracellular activation, 31–32
Intrapancreatic duct activation, 32
Intravascular volume, 67–68
Intrinsic factor, 118
Ischemia, 35, 38, 68

J

Jaundice, 173–174
Juvenile idiopathic pancreatitis, 110

K

Kallikrein, 29
Kallikreinogen, 3
Kazal inhibitor, 3
Kwashiorkor, 43

L

Labeled-lipid tests, 118–119
Lactic acidosis, 93
Lactoferrin, 5, 116
Laparotomy, 47, 76

Lesions, 108
  detection of, 161–162
Lindau's disease, 157
Lipase, 1, 29–31, 94
  diagnosis and, 50–51
  malabsorption and, 135–137
Lipolytic enzymes, 3–4
Lundh test, 115
Lysolecithin, 4
Lysosomal enzymes, 4–5

M

Macroamylasemia, 51
Magnesium, 96–97
Magnetic resonance imaging, 61
Malabsorption, 24, 173
  in chronic pancreatitis, 101
  management of, 135–137
Malnutritional pancreatitis, 43, 99, 108–109
Masses, 125–127
  detection of, 162
Meal-stimulation test, 115
Meconium ileus, 146–147
Melena, 106
Meperidine, 67, 134
6-Mercaptopurine, 39
Mesotrypsinogen, 2
Metabolic abnormalities, 91–94
Metabolic diseases, 41–42
Metastatic status, 170–171
Methemalbumin, 52, 54
Methyldopa, 40
Migrating motility complex, 12
Mitomycin-C, 177
MMC, see Migrating motility complex
Monitor peptide, 20
Morphine, 19, 67, 134
Mortality rates
  abscess, 74
  acute pancreatitis, 55
  chronic pancreatitis, 107
  injury, 84
  necrotic pseudocysts, 103
  pancreatic ascites, 81
  surgery, 138, 141, 171
Motilin, 12
Muscarinic receptors, 16

N

Narcotics, 134
NBT-PABA (Bentiromide) test, 117
Necrotic pseudocysts, 103
Necrotizing pancreatitis, 24
  abscess and, 73
Neoplasms, 76, 165
Nerves, 100–101, 133–135, 175
Neural mechanisms, 15–21

INDEX

Neurofibromatosis, 157
Neuropeptide Y, 19
Neurotensin, 17–18
Nodal status, 170–171
Noninvasive tests, 116–120

O

Obstructive chronic pancreatitis, 24, 99, 109
Oleic acid, 19
Oligosaccharides, 4
Omeprazole, 137
Opiates, 19, 67
Oxidation, 35
Oxycodone, 134

P

Palliation, 173–175
Pancreas divisum, 37, 57–58, 144
Pancreatic ascites, 78–83
Pancreatic insufficiency, 147–149
Pancreatic juice, 1–5
 analysis of, 116
 collection of, 114–115
Pancreaticoduodenectomy, 84, 140
Pancreaticojejunostomy, 138, 171
Pancreatic polypeptide (PP), 12, 14, 18, 120
Pancreatic stone protein (PSP), 5, 36, 166
Pancreatitis, 23; see also Acute pancreatitis;
 Chronic pancreatitis
Pancreolauryl test, 117–118
Para-amino benzoic (PABA), 117
Parasites, 37
Pathogenic mechanisms, 29–44
Pentazocine, 134
Peptic ulcers, 43, 106–107
Peptidergic pathways, 13
Peptides, stimulatory, 114
Peptide YY, 19
Percutaneous drainage, 74, 77–78, 133
Peristaltic activity, 12
Peritoneal lavage, 71, 74, 84
Pharynx, 13
Phospholipase A_2, 1, 4, 29–31
 inhibitors, 71
Phosphorus, 97
Plasmin, 32
Pleural effusions, 88, 106
Polarity, 7
Porphyria, 44
Postoperative pancreatitis, 40–41
 abscess and, 73
Potassium, 97
PP, see Pancreatic polypeptide
Propoxyphene, 134
Proteases, 1, 134
Protein plug hypothesis, 35–36

Proteins, 1
 biosynthesis of, 9–10
 nonenzyme, 116
 R, 118
 serum, 5
Proteolytic enzymes, 1–3
Pruritus, 173
Pseudoaneurysms, 106
Pseudocysts, 24, 75–79, 129
 acute pancreatitis and, 27
 chronic pancreatitis and, 100, 102–104
 treatment of, 132–133
PSP, see Pancreatic stone protein
Pulmonary complications, 88–90

R

Radiation, 175–177
Radioimmunoassay (RIA), 51–52
Radiology
 acute pancreatitis and, 61–65
 cancer and, 161–169
 chronic pancreatitis and, 125–129
Ras oncogenes, 157
Receptors, 7
Renal complications, 90
Renal disease, 44
Renal failure, 96–97
Renal transplant, 42
Resection, 139–141, 175
 cancer and, 171
Respiratory tract, 31
 cystic fibrosis and, 147
 failure, 88–89
Retention pseudocysts, 104
Reye syndrome, 150
RIA, see Radioimmunoassay
Ribonucleases, 3
Rough ER membrane, 9

S

Salivary amylase, 4
Sarcomas, 175
Scorpion venom poisoning, 42–43
Secretagogues, 7–9
Secretin, 11, 16, 114–116
Secretin-CCK test, 115, 122
Secretion, 12–15
 control of, 11–15
 rate of, 1
 suppression of, 69–72
 testing for cancer, 161
Secretory cells, 5–11
Senile idiopathic pancreatitis, 110
Sepsis, 89–90
Serous cystadenomas, 165
Serum
 amylase concentration, 49, 53

INDEX

Serum (contd.)
  fluorescein, 117–118
  lipase, 50–51
  testing for cancer, 160–161
  trypsinogen, 119–120
Shock, 38, 68
Shwachman-Diamond syndrome, 144, 148–149
Smoking, 11, 107
  cancer and, 155–157
Sodium, 11
Sodium bicarbonate, 136
Somatostatin, 18–19, 70, 82
Sonography, 61–65
  cancer and, 161–163
  chronic pancreatitis and, 125
Soybean trypsin inhibitor, 2
Spectrophotometric method, 51
Sphincter of Oddi, 38, 57
Sphincterotomy, 56–57, 128
Steatorrhea, 3, 24, 137
  in chronic pancreatitis, 101
Stents, 57
  cancer and, 167–168
  chronic pancreatitis and, 128–129
  jaundice and, 174
Steroids, 40, 150
Stimulation, direct, 114–115
Stimulus-secretion coupling, 7
Stomach, 14
Stools, 119
  chymotrypsinogen in, 120
  in cystic fibrosis, 146–147
Stress ulcers, 91, 105
Sulfonamides, 39
Surgery, 40–41
  abscess and, 74–75
  cancer and, 171–173
  chronic pancreatitis and, 137–141
  injury and, 84
  jaundice and, 174
  pseudocyst and, 76–77
Sweat test, 149–150

T

Tetracycline, 40
Thrombin, 32
Thrombosis, 29, 90
  splenic vein, 105–106
Thyrotropin-releasing hormone (TRH), 14

Titrimetric method, 51
Transfusions, 68
Transition, 9–10
Trauma, 41, 57, 83–85, 150
Triglycerides, 41–42
  cystic fibrosis and, 148
  test with, 118–119
Triolein breath test, 118
Tropical pancreatitis, 43, 99, 108–109
Trypsin, 29–33
  feedback and, 20
Trypsinogen, 1–2, 34
  diagnosis and, 51
  serum, 119–120
Trypsin-trypsin inhibitor ratio, 36
Tumor markers, 116
Tumor Node Metastasis (TNM) Classification, 169–171
Tumors, benign, 157–158
Tumor status, 170–171
Turbidimetric method, 51

U

Ultrasound, 64
  cancer and, 161–163
  chronic pancreatitis and, 127–129
  injury and, 84
  pseudocyst and, 76
Urinary amylase excretion, 49
Urine, 117–120

V

Vagal cholinergic pathways, 13
Vagotomy, 13–14, 171
Valproic acid, 40
Vascular damage, 29
Vasoactive intestinal peptide (VIP), 17–18
Vitamins, 101
  B-12, 118
  cystic fibrosis and, 148

W

Water, 7, 11
  alcohol and, 36
Whipple pancreaticoduodenectomy, 139–140, 171

Z

Zymogen granules, 9–10, 27, 31